About the End Sheets

The limestone blocks in the two lowest floors of the Plummer Building's exterior offer a fascinating mix of artistic surprises. Look up as you walk by and you'll discover a sprinkling of mythological and allegorical themes beautifully displayed in bas-relief on the walls of the historic building.

A variety of animals and birds share space with people and objects meaningful to patients, employees, and friends of Mayo Clinic. For example, Saint George (patron saint of England, the birthplace of Dr. William Worrall Mayo) appears on the wall, slaying a dragon. There's a trimotor airplane, the type of aircraft first to land in Rochester. You'll see a motorboat on a Minnesota lake, a corncob, a Viking ship, even a hunched-over Dr. Henry Plummer, scrutinizing the building's architectural drawings.

The sheets at the beginning and end of this book record Jack Desley's drawings of some of these interesting, thought-provoking carvings. You'll also find them within the text, just as Dr. Plummer randomly positioned the carvings on the building. They convey both the genius and the humor of the pioneering Mayo physician for whom the building is named.

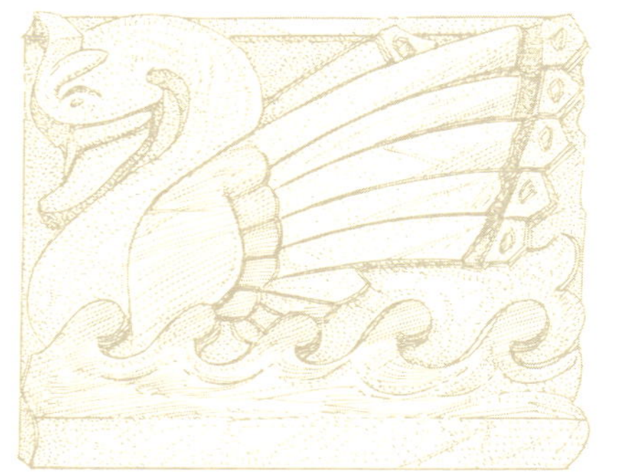
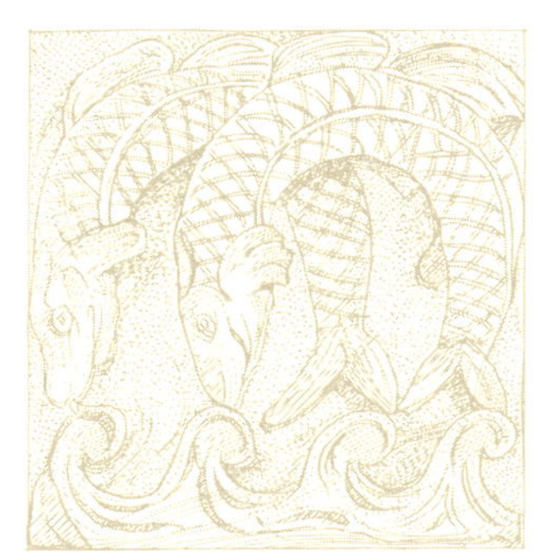
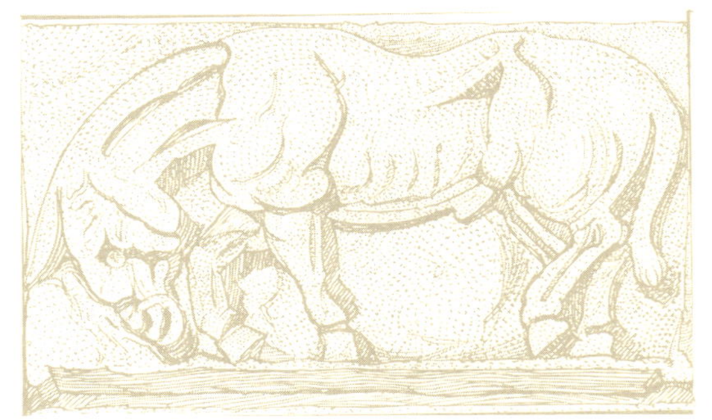
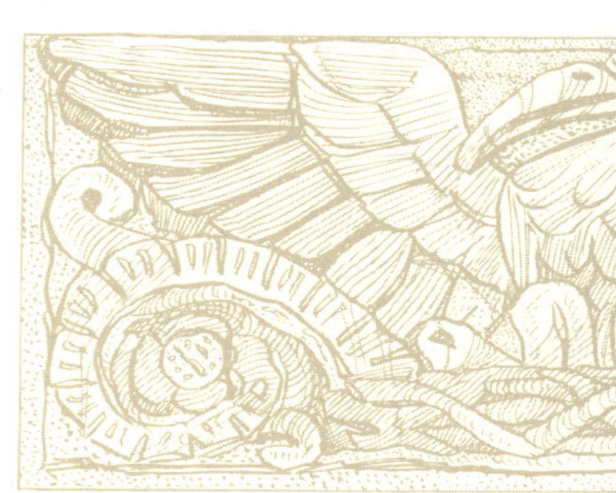

Foreword

The professional staff of Mayo Clinic was fortunate to have available for many years the artistic skills and the cheerful cooperation of John W. Desley. When he joined the Mayo staff, he was already a medical illustrator with educational and experience credentials of a high order. John quickly, but quietly, demonstrated his capacity to contribute in a major way to the extensive publication and educational endeavors of the Mayo staff.

A longtime member (still current) of the Association of Medical Illustrators, John served that organization as a member of its Board of Governors for five years. Clearly, his expertise and dedication have been recognized by his peers nationally as well as by those in Rochester.

John Desley's drawings provide an interesting and attractive perspective on the evolution of Mayo Clinic. His views of Mayo's growth reflect the endless increase in physical facilities required to accommodate the steady increases in the scope and nature of Mayo's professional endeavors.

In the beginning, the Mayo enterprise was an office/outcall practice of Dr. William Worrall Mayo and his two sons, Drs. William James and Charles Horace Mayo. When Saint Marys Hospital offered beds and an operating room, the practice grew rapidly. Physician partners and associates were added and the concept of a coordinated group practice developed, housed in the first Mayo Clinic building (see page 55).

Formal programs in education and research generated new space needs. After World War II, Mayo Clinic grew to become a comprehensive medical center with clinical, educational and research activities occupying a sizable medical campus. In the past decade, the growth of Mayo Clinic Jacksonville and Mayo Clinic Scottsdale and numerous affiliations with physicians and hospitals within 100 miles or so of Rochester suggest that the Mayo enterprise is now a Health Care System.

The Desley drawings provide a pictorial record of this amazing Mayo history. The people of Mayo and you who enjoy this book are indebted to John for his deep interest in Mayo, his keen selection of Mayo vistas, and his considerable effort in creating this collection for our pleasure.

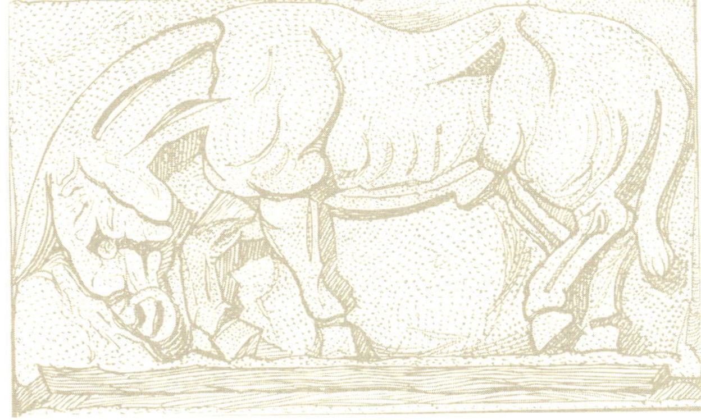

Robert C. Roesler
Chair Emeritus, Department of Administration
Member Emeritus, Board of Governors and Board of Trustees, Mayo Foundation,
Rochester, Minnesota

This book is dedicated

to the women and men of Mayo Clinic

Preface and Acknowledgments

The drawings in this book were done mostly on my own time over the span of my career as a Mayo Clinic medical illustrator. I could not have created this series without the encouragement and devotion of my wife of 42 years, Janice Reed Desley, who also was an artist. All of our six children have careers in medicine or art. Janice died three years ago. I've since been blessed with a new bride, Margaret Wakeman. Margaret is the second guiding light for my artistic endeavors, which continue now from our log home in North Carolina.

My friend David Pennington deserves much credit for this book. Dave gathered a sampling of my drawings and drafted captions. He asked Mayo Medical Ventures to consider publishing this material. Kevin Hennessey, director of the Medical Products Division of Mayo Medical Ventures, liked the concept and, together with James Marttila, a member of his staff, moved it forward, gaining required approvals and endorsements and gathering the drawings.

Special thanks to my friend Robert Roesler, Chair Emeritus of the Mayo Clinic Department of Administration and a former member of our Board of Governors and Board of Trustees, for skillfully crafting the foreword for this book. Through the years, Bob played a major role in the establishment and nurture of Mayo's expansive art program. He personally coordinated acquisition and placement of many of the wonderful objects of art that grace the sides, plazas, and interiors of Mayo Clinic buildings.

Special thanks also go to Dr. Carolyn Beck, Nicole Babcock, and Clark Nelson for carefully reviewing the text for factual accuracy and for providing reference material. Dr. Beck is coordinator of the Mayo Center for Humanities in Medicine and the Mayo Historical Suite. Nicole Babcock is Dr. Beck's knowledgeable associate. Mr. Nelson, author of *Mayo Roots: Profiling the Origins of Mayo Clinic,* for more than 30 years served as Mayo's historical archivist. I also want to thank the Olmsted County Historical Society for assistance with research, and Robert Benassi, Matthew Dacy, Richard Edwards, Thomas Hamer, Marianne Hockema, Michael Homan, Marvin Mitchell, Joel Rueber, Nancy Skaran, Robert Tryggestad, and Kim Van Nimwegen for assistance with information and fact checking.

The art director for this book was Patricia Boyd, whose experience and expertise in graphic design are evident on every page and on the book's attractive jacket. Editorial production was coordinated by LeAnn Stee, who so ably heads the Mayo Section of Publications. Suzanne Leaf-Brock, of the Mayo Division of Communications, planned and managed marketing efforts. Joseph Liesse, manager of The Mayo Store, supervised distribution, sales, and customer service. Jonathan Bedsted coordinated printing and mechanical production. David Swanson, editor-at-large in Mayo Medical Ventures, was managing editor. The book was printed by Davies Printing Company, Rochester, Minnesota.

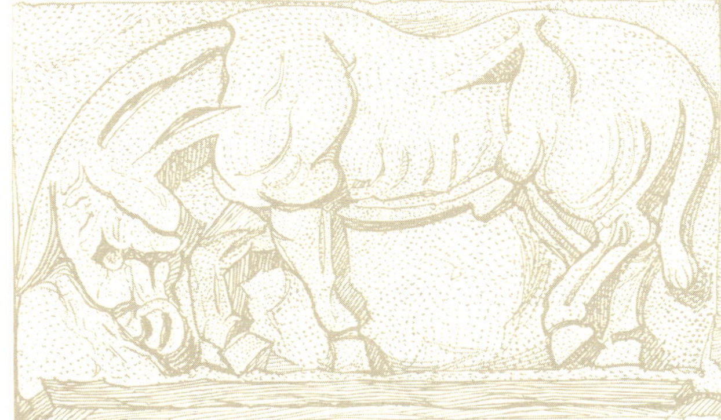

Most of all, I want to express appreciation to my former employer, Mayo Clinic. I have the utmost respect and affection for the renowned medical center that enabled me to create not only medical illustrations that contribute to the worldwide advancement of scientific knowledge but also artistic works of lasting beauty and worth.

John W. Desley

Contents

Artist's Overview

Winslow Homer told a story about a gentleman who walked up to him once as he was working on a watercolor painting. Said the gentleman: "How long does it take you to do a painting like this?" Homer's reply: "About 40 years."

That story stuck in my mind. An artist never stops learning. Everything you've done in the past contributes to the results of whatever it is you happen to be working on. And every drawing or painting you finish has a life of its own. If you are creating something beautiful, unique, or worthwhile, there's never a time limit to its usefulness. It may be destroyed but it won't "wear out," and you can never really know how your work might affect viewers.

The first drawing I did for the series in this book was the closing of the bronze doors of the Plummer Building. Several additional views of the splendid building followed. I hadn't realized just how important these drawings would be until I received a phone call one day from a patient at Rochester Methodist Hospital.

Daisy Plummer, wife of Dr. Henry Plummer, the Mayo Clinic physician whose name the Plummer Building bears, was on the line. She seemed to be quite ill but made a special effort to pick up the phone and tell me my drawings of the Plummer Building gave her comfort. She asked if I would I please have three drawings framed and sent to her hospital room as soon as possible. She wanted them hung on the wall at the foot of her bed.

Mrs. Plummer especially wanted to view my drawing of the closing of the Plummer Building doors (see page 7). Later I recalled the doors had been ceremoniously closed on the passing of her husband. I was touched by her request and proud that I had created something of such special value to the wife of one of our pioneering Mayo Clinic physicians. The drawings were hung. Mrs. Plummer died a week later.

The third drawing in this series is the view of the Plummer Building bell tower (see page 9), which prominently includes Canadian geese in graceful V formations. Each autumn, thousands of these majestic birds flock to Rochester where they spend their winter months lounging in Silver Lake, which is warmed by clean waste water from a local electrical power plant.

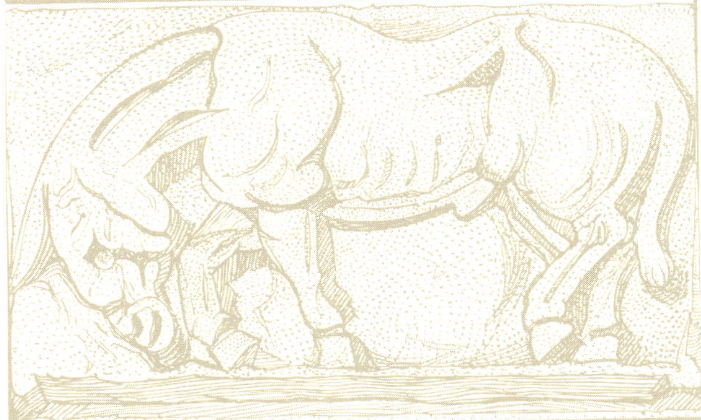

At the time I began thinking about drawing the bell tower, I'd signed on with Mayo but still lived in Minneapolis. Each morning I commuted to Rochester by air. The airport is situated several miles south of the city, so it meant a daily bus ride to town and to my office in the Plummer Building.

Our bus and those big birds seemed to be on the same early morning travel schedule. Daily we were escorted into town by multiple formations of geese. They had dined and spent the night in cornfields near the airport and were heading for Silver Lake, a mile north of Mayo Clinic, to meet friends, make new acquaintances, and begin their day of collective honking, wing flapping, bobbing beneath the water for snacks, and carrying on as geese do all day long on our little city-bound lake.

One morning, as we approached the Mayo Clinic complex downtown, the sky around the Plummer Building bell tower was filled with geese. The scene was imprinted on my mind as I sketched this drawing, which blends the glory and majesty of the Plummer Building's ornate architecture with the simplicity, strength, and beauty of these remarkable feathered residents of our town.

As I look back on the pen-and-ink drawings I've done through the years, pleasant memories flood my mind. Behind each drawing, there's a story. I enjoy reflecting on these recollections, especially when they involve people who own my work.

Once I was asked to draw Supreme Court Justice Harry Blackmun who, before moving from Rochester to Washington, D. C., was employed as our Mayo Clinic legal counsel. Through the years, Justice Blackmun has nurtured his Rochester roots, returning now and then for business or social purposes and occasionally to address Mayo physicians and administrators on topics of mutual interest.

I decided to draw Justice Blackmun in action on one of these occasions. The setting was Balfour Hall, on the third floor of Mayo Foundation House. Mayo Foundation House is the former home of Dr. and Mrs. William J. Mayo (see page 43).

Balfour Hall is an elegant, spacious room that was used by the Mayos for entertaining, mainly dancing. The Mayos designed their home to be an extension of Mayo Clinic facilities, often hosting parties for visiting medical and political dignitaries, sometimes putting them up overnight. After living in the home for 20 years, Dr. and Mrs. Mayo donated it to Mayo Foundation for use as a meeting place where people in medicine can exchange ideas "for the good of mankind." Balfour Hall became the room of choice for occasions such as a talk by a Supreme Court Justice.

I should point out that Justice Blackmun is every bit as distinguished in appearance as in his record of public service. He has a full head of curly gray hair, a chiseled visage, and piercing eyes that arrest attention and demand respect. So I had these traits going for me as I began to sketch the drawing.

The setting in Balfour Hall also was a plus. The hall features a huge stained-glass window. The rest of the cathedral-beamed room is paneled with wood stained dark brown. It's a beautiful room. I included some of this majestic architecture in the drawing. The piece was framed and sent to Justice Blackmun's office at the Supreme Court in Washington, D. C.

A week later a postal worker marched into my office carrying a white envelope with Justice Blackmun's name and Supreme Court address in the upper left corner. The hand-delivered envelope contained a warm letter of thanks from Justice Blackmun, who wanted to convey special appreciation for what I'd recorded with pen, ink, and paper.

Unique gestures of appreciation from people of international stature are day brighteners. But so are the words, notes, and simple expressions of thanks from individuals in all walks of life who are touched in some special way by my work. Such sentiments make my life more meaningful and worthwhile.

I hope you'll appreciate the drawings selected for this book as much as I've enjoyed working with the people who commissioned them, the process behind the creation of each piece, and the sentiments of people who view and display them for others to enjoy.

John W. Desley

John W. Desley
Lewisville, North Carolina

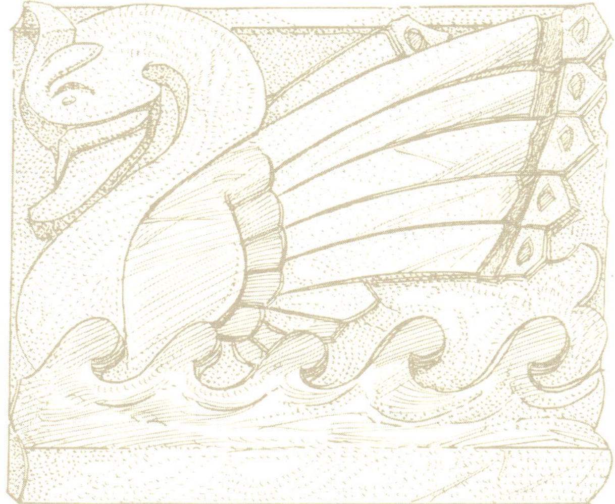

Plummer Building Doors *(Open)*

(Plate 1)

The ornate entrance to the Plummer Building features two sets of doors. Both were designed to be closed at the end of each Clinic day. In practice, the two-ton, 16-foot-high, solid bronze outer doors are closed only for special, ceremonial occasions.

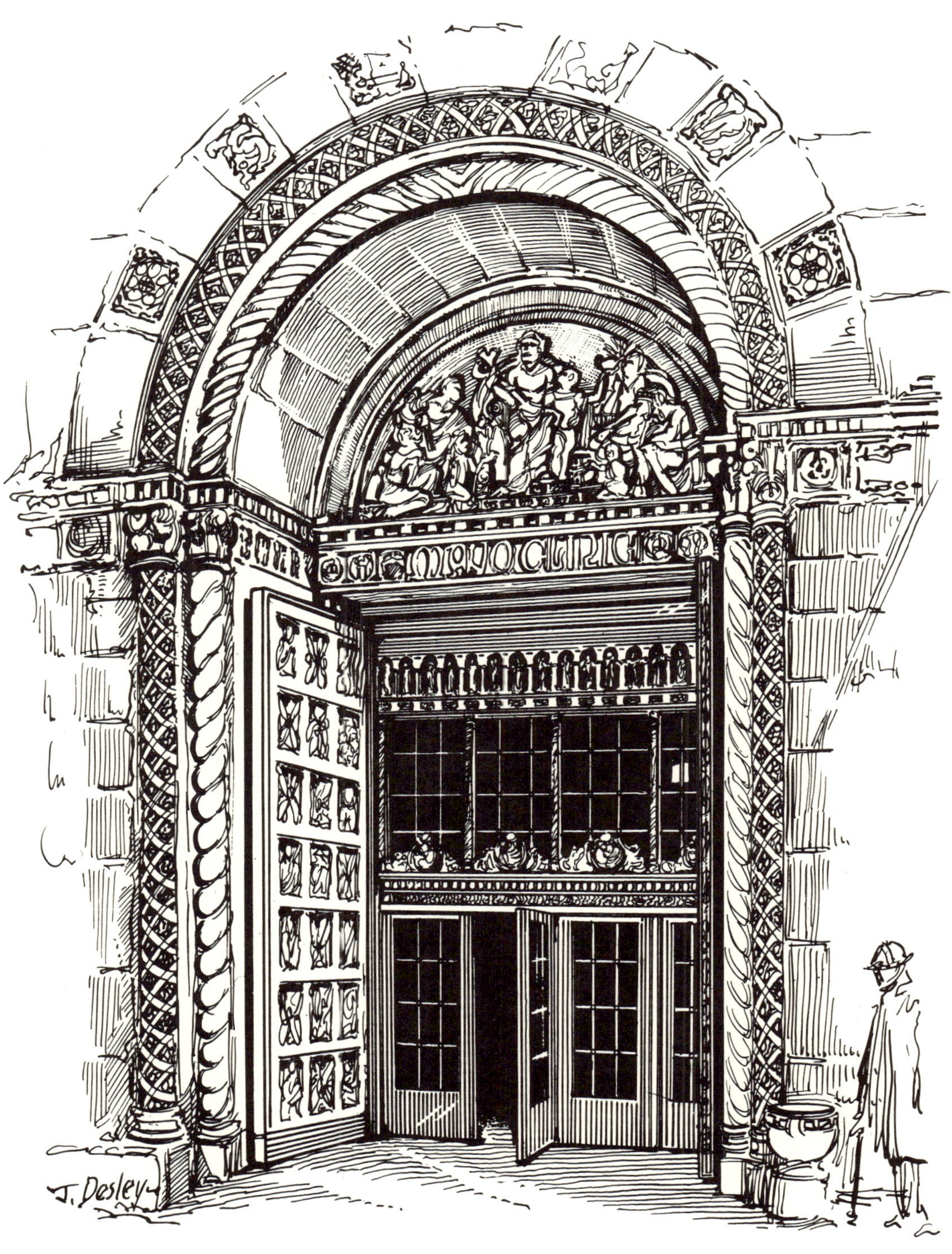

(Plate 1)

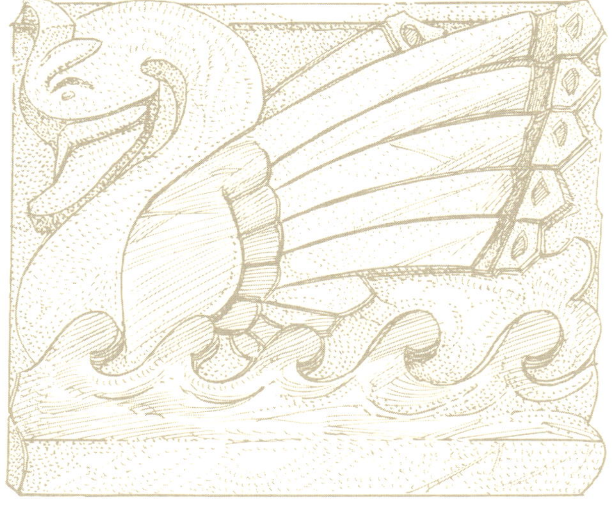

"Mrs. Plummer made a special effort to pick up the phone and tell me my drawings of the Plummer Building gave her comfort. I was touched by her request and proud that I had created something of such special value to the wife of one of our pioneering Mayo Clinic physicians."—JWD

Plummer Building Doors *(Closed)*

(Plate 2)

Only a few times has death closed the great bronze doors of the Plummer Building. Although records are incomplete, ceremonial closings are believed to have occurred upon the deaths of Drs. E. Starr Judd, Henry S. Plummer, William J. Mayo, Charles H. Mayo, Charles W. Mayo, and Donald C. Balfour. The doors were also closed for Harry J. Harwick, longtime business administrator at Mayo Clinic, and for the assassinated 35th President of the United States, John F. Kennedy.

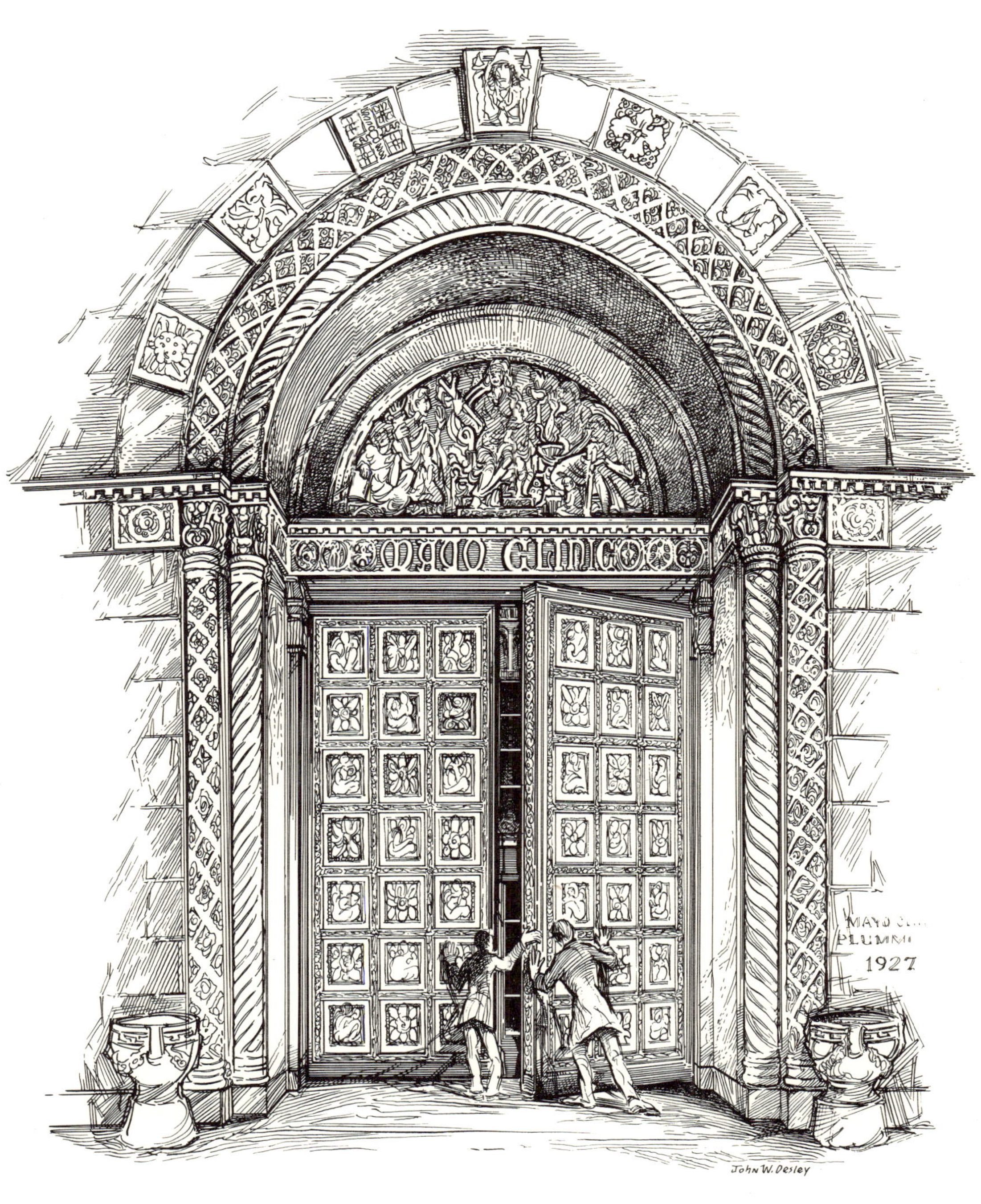

(Plate 2)

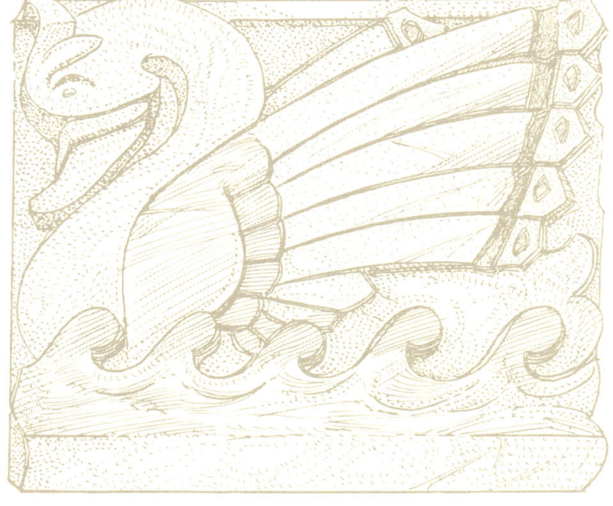

"One morning, as we approached the Mayo Clinic complex downtown, the sky around the Plummer Building bell tower was filled with geese. The scene was imprinted on my mind as I sketched this drawing, which blends the glory and majesty of the Plummer Building's ornate architecture with the simplicity, strength, and beauty of these remarkable feathered residents of our town."—JWD

Plummer Building Bell Tower

(Plate 3)

For almost 70 years, the familiar bell tower atop this building has stood as a beacon of healing and hope for Mayo Clinic patients. The building was named for Dr. Henry S. Plummer, the early Mayo physician who conceived the system of an integrated medical group practice that the building served. Working with the architectural firm of Ellerbe & Company, Dr. Plummer coordinated the building's design and construction. The building opened in 1928. It housed most of the outpatient practice until 1953, when a new clinical facility opened and the older structure was renamed in honor of Dr. Plummer. The tower houses the 56-bell Rochester Carillon.

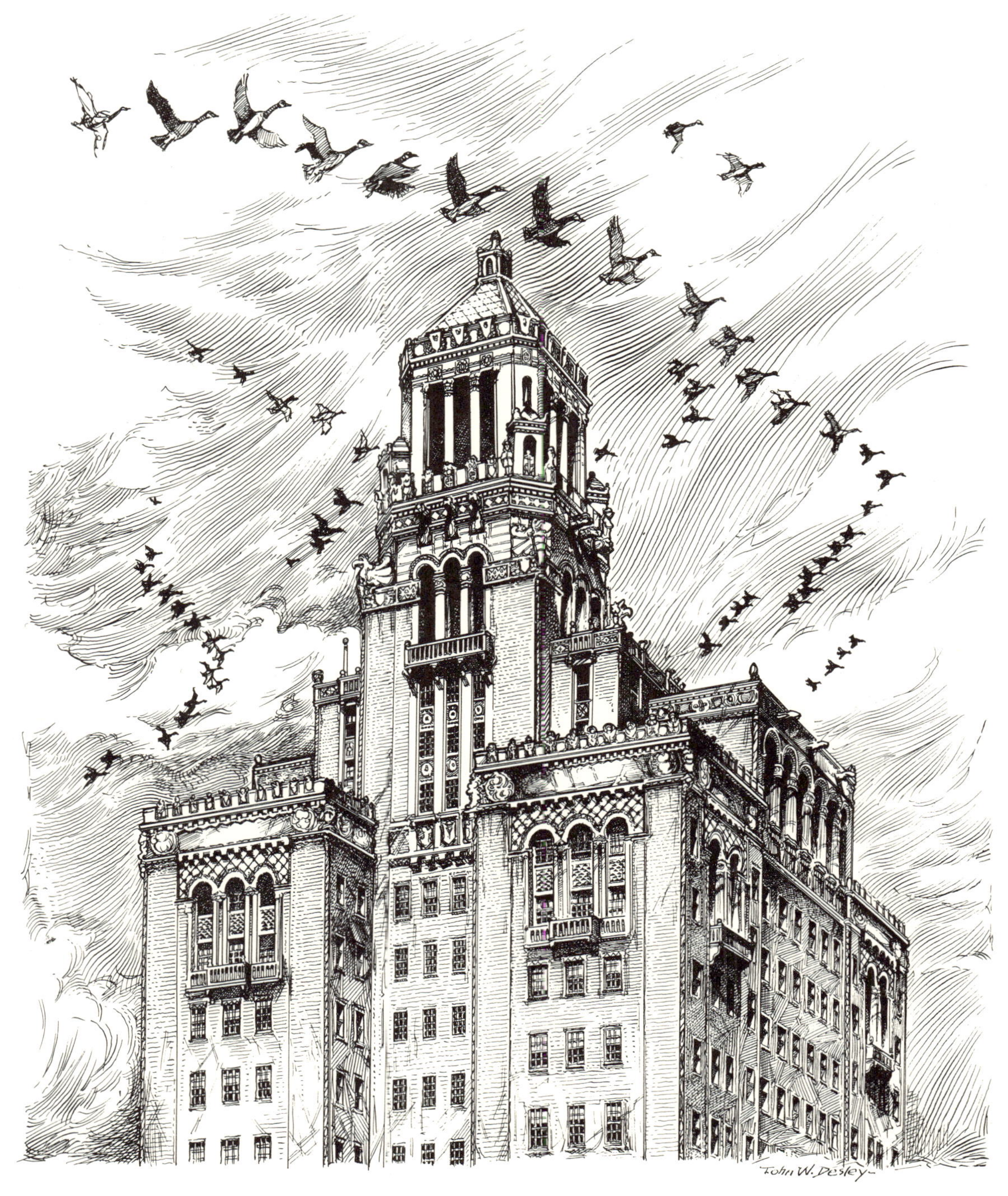

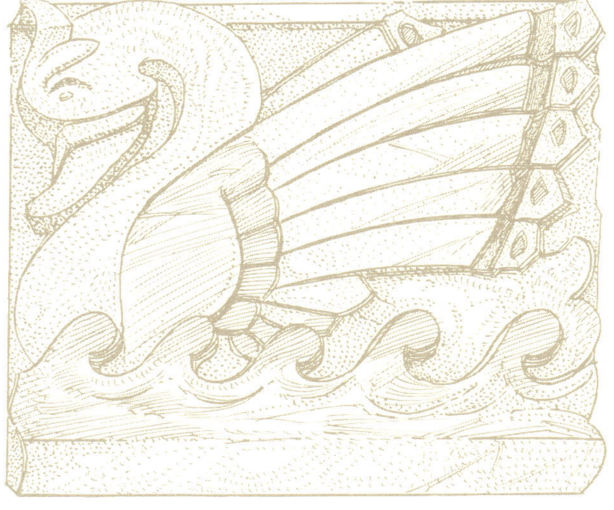

"The original Board of Governors' Room is one of the most impressive and popular historic sites on the Mayo Rochester campus. The craftsmanship of the builders is evident from floor to ceiling, but the wall hangings, detailing the remarkable accomplishments of the Mayo brothers, are what draw people into the room and keep them there, sometimes for extended periods."—JWD

Board of Governors' Room

(Plate 4)

Earned and honorary degrees, titles, certificates, honors, and awards cover three walls of the original Board of Governors' room on the third floor of the Plummer Building. The framed citations document the remarkable accomplishments and international reputations of Drs. William J. and Charles H. Mayo, who founded Mayo Clinic. A delicate, open, lace-like colored ceiling and stained-glass windows are other features of the room, which is open weekdays for public tours.

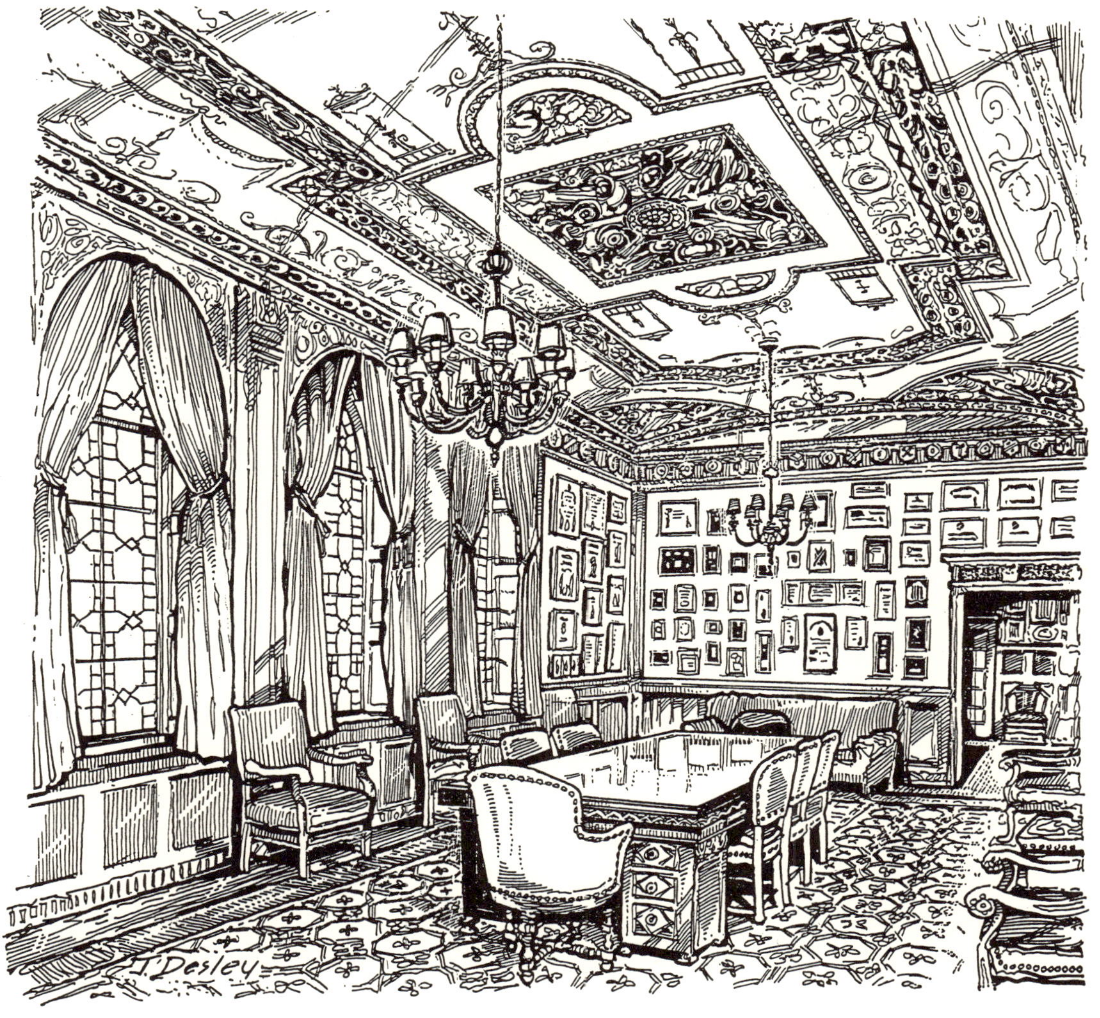

(Plate 4)

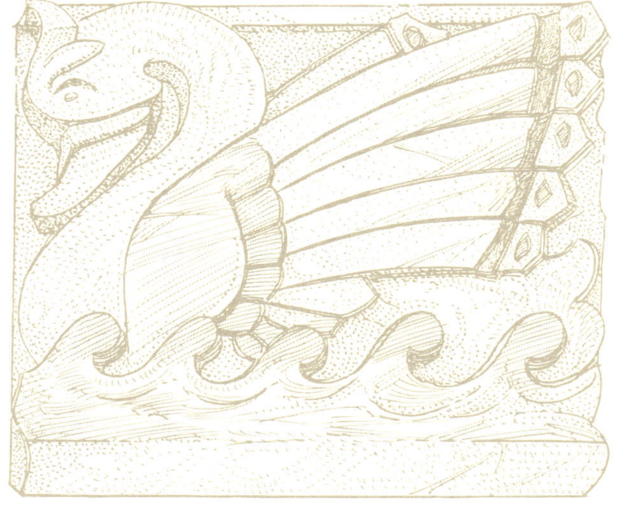

"This drawing depicts one very impressive room of the library as it appeared in the 1930s. Although some of the furnishings have changed, the ceiling, light fixtures, windows, and walls remain essentially unaltered."—JWD

Mayo Medical Library

(Plate 5)

Carved and painted wood beams on the ceiling of Mayo Hall in Mayo Medical Library name many of medicine's greatest contributors. Dr. Plummer personally selected the names of those cited on the ceiling beams. The library occupies five floors of the Plummer Building. More than 350,000 volumes and over 4,000 current subscriptions to medical and scientific journals are available for use by Mayo physicians, scientists, and allied-health staff members. The library's on-line catalog offers electronic access to medical journals and literature worldwide. The library was established in 1907. In 1909, it moved into a small, red-brick building on the northeast corner of the Plummer Building location. Later it occupied the third floor of the 1914 Mayo Clinic building (see page 55) before moving into the Plummer Building. This spacious room, on the 12th floor, houses the circulation desk and other services.

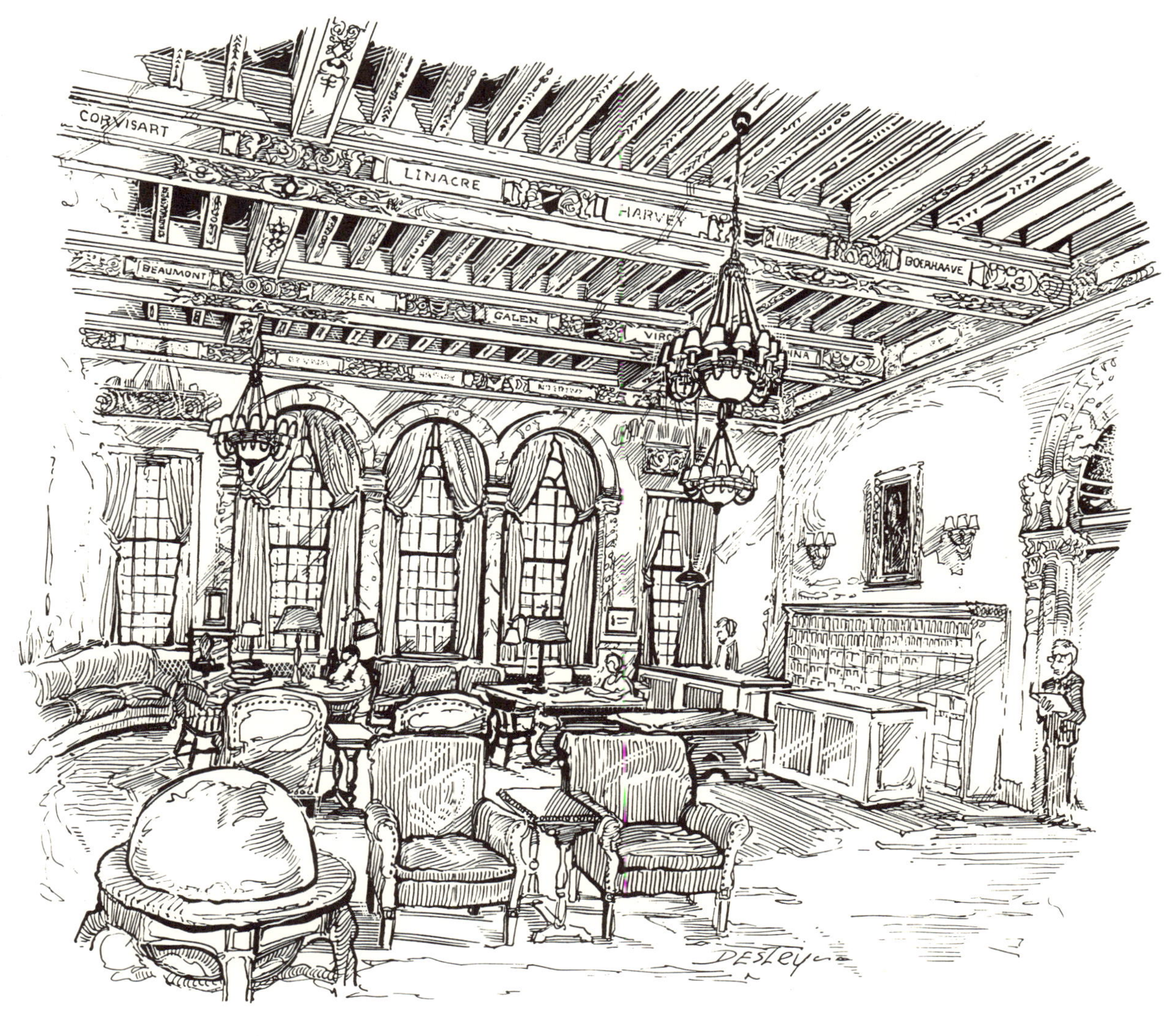
CORVISART
LINACRE
HARVEY
BEAUMONT
BOERHAAVE
GALEN
DESLEY

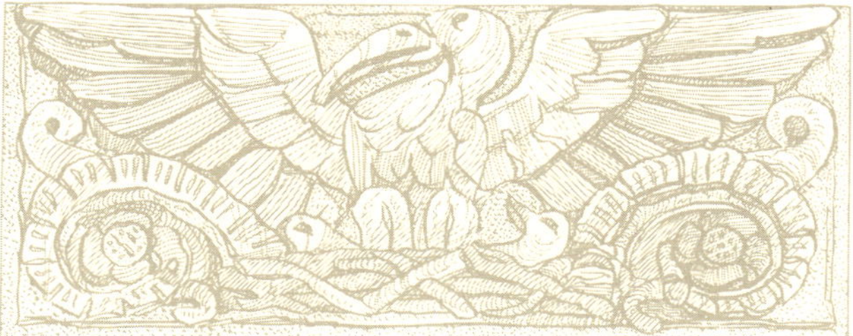

Mayo Building ***(Northeast Facade)***

(Plate 6)

The white and gray Georgia marble Mayo Building is the primary outpatient diagnostic facility of Mayo Clinic Rochester. Ellerbe & Company was the architect. The building represents an advancement of interior design concepts and operational systems established by Dr. Henry Plummer to facilitate the integrated group practice of medicine that was pioneered in the building that now bears his name (see page 9). The first ten floors of the Mayo Building were completed in 1955. By 1969, the building had grown another nine floors to stretch almost 300 feet into the sky. Murals, paintings, photographs, and other objects of art grace interior walls and lobbies of the building. Sculptures are positioned in plazas and on north, south, and east facades. A large telecommunications dish is positioned on the roof to facilitate telemedicine and educational and administrative teleconferences, primarily with Mayo facilities in Jacksonville, Florida, and Scottsdale, Arizona.

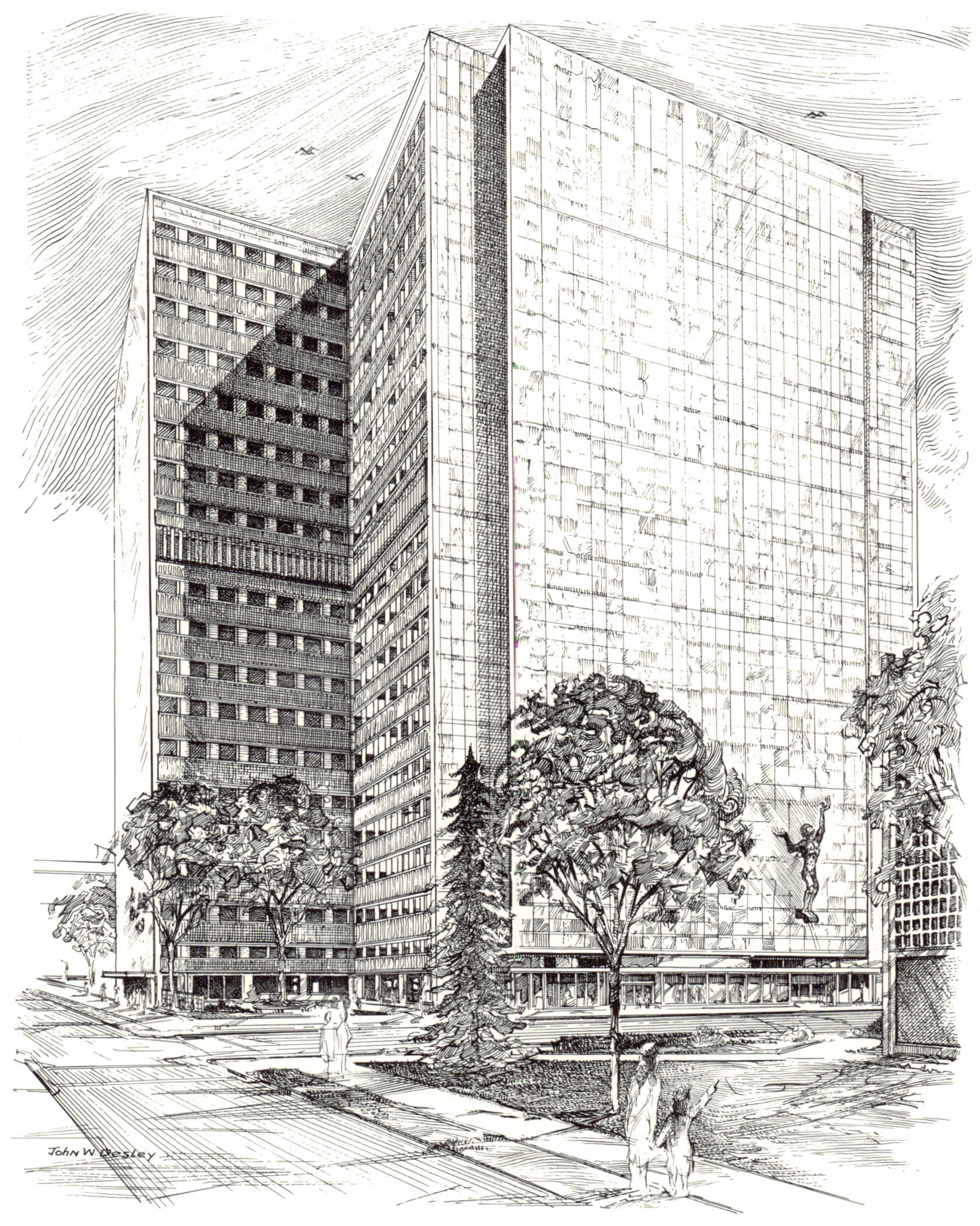
John W. Desley

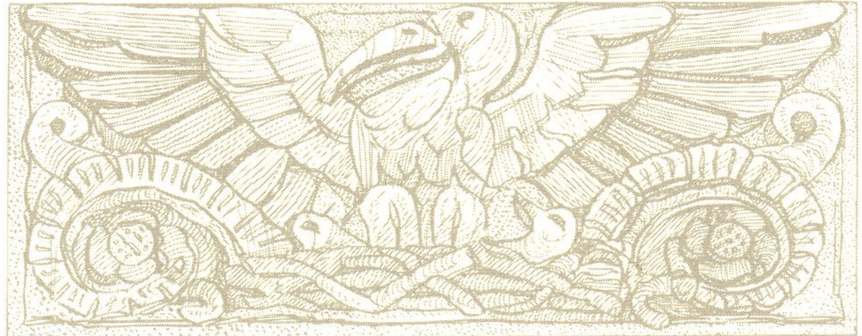

"I was intrigued by the relationship of the old to the new in this classic perspective of our clinical facilities."—JWD

Mayo and Plummer Buildings

(Plate 7)

Mayo Building, left, and Plummer Building, right, are familiar landmarks of the Rochester Mayo downtown medical complex. This view features the southwest facades of the buildings.

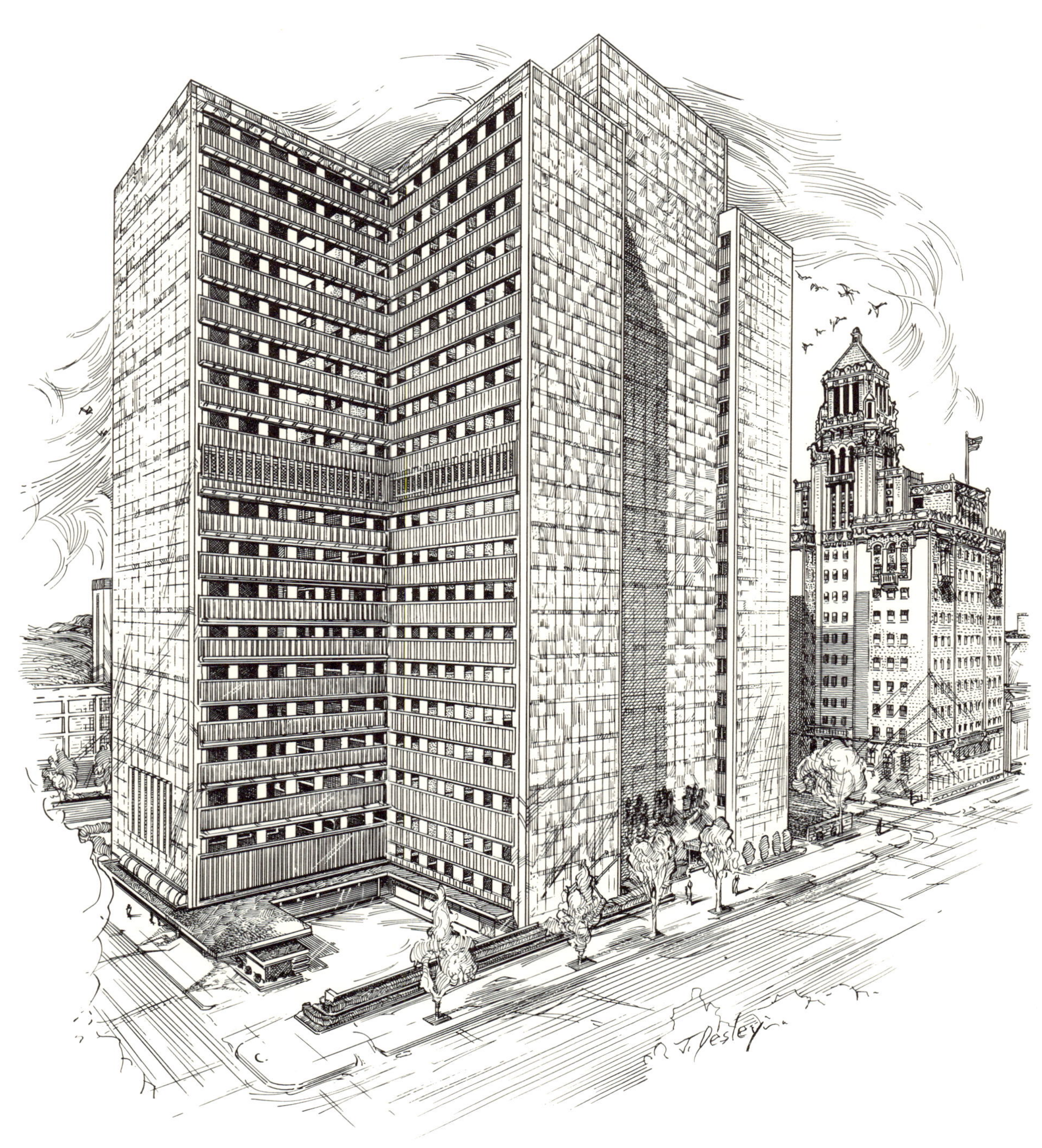

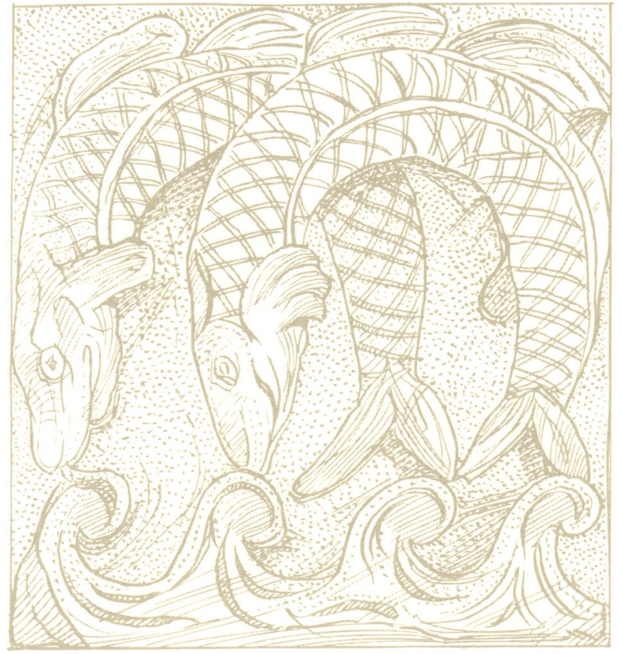

"This drawing was originally used as background art for the first Mayo Medical School diploma."—JWD

Mitchell Student Center ***(Mayo Medical School)***

(Plate 8)

The Ruth and Frederick Mitchell Student Center of Mayo Medical School honors Mayo benefactor Ruth M. Masson and her first husband, Frederick M. Mitchell. The building, for 30 years home to the Rochester Public Library, was built in 1936-37 under the aegis of the Federal Public Works Administration. It was later purchased by Mayo Foundation. Mayo Medical School, founded in 1972, is recognized nationally for excellence. Annually the school receives nearly 4,000 applications for 40 openings in the first-year class. Total enrollment, including students engaged in Mayo's MD/PhD program, is approximately 180.

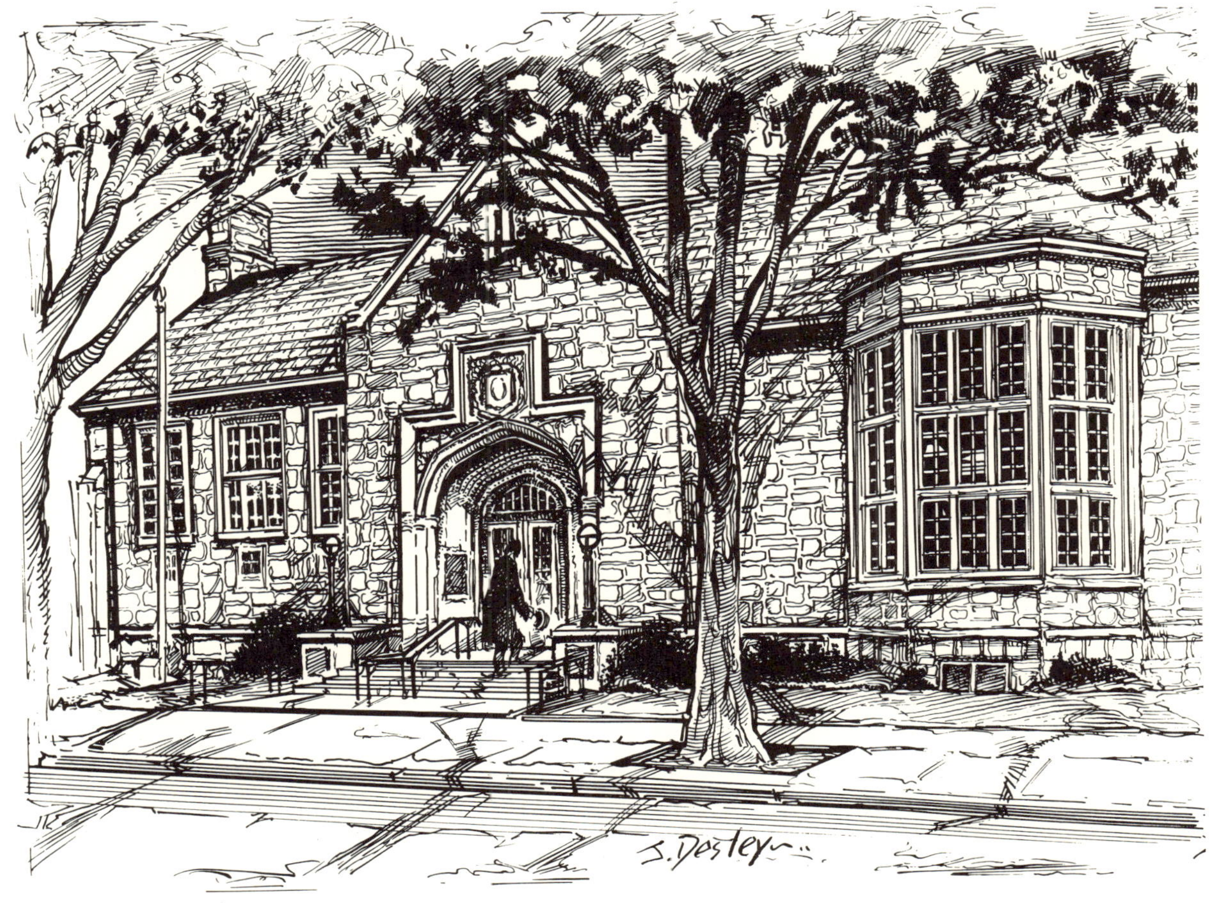

(Plate 8)

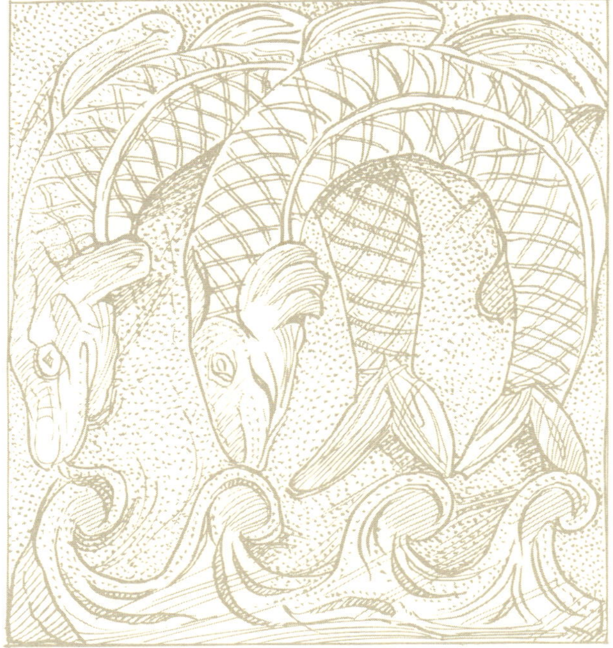

Mitchell Student Center Entrance

(Plate 9)

This closeup view of the front entrance to the Mitchell Student Center of Mayo Medical School captures the essence and elegance of the little building, considered by some to be an "architectural gem" nestled among taller contemporary Mayo structures (see page 39). The building was designed by Harold H. Crawford, a prominent Rochester area architect. It was renovated and dedicated as the Student Center of Mayo Medical School in 1985.

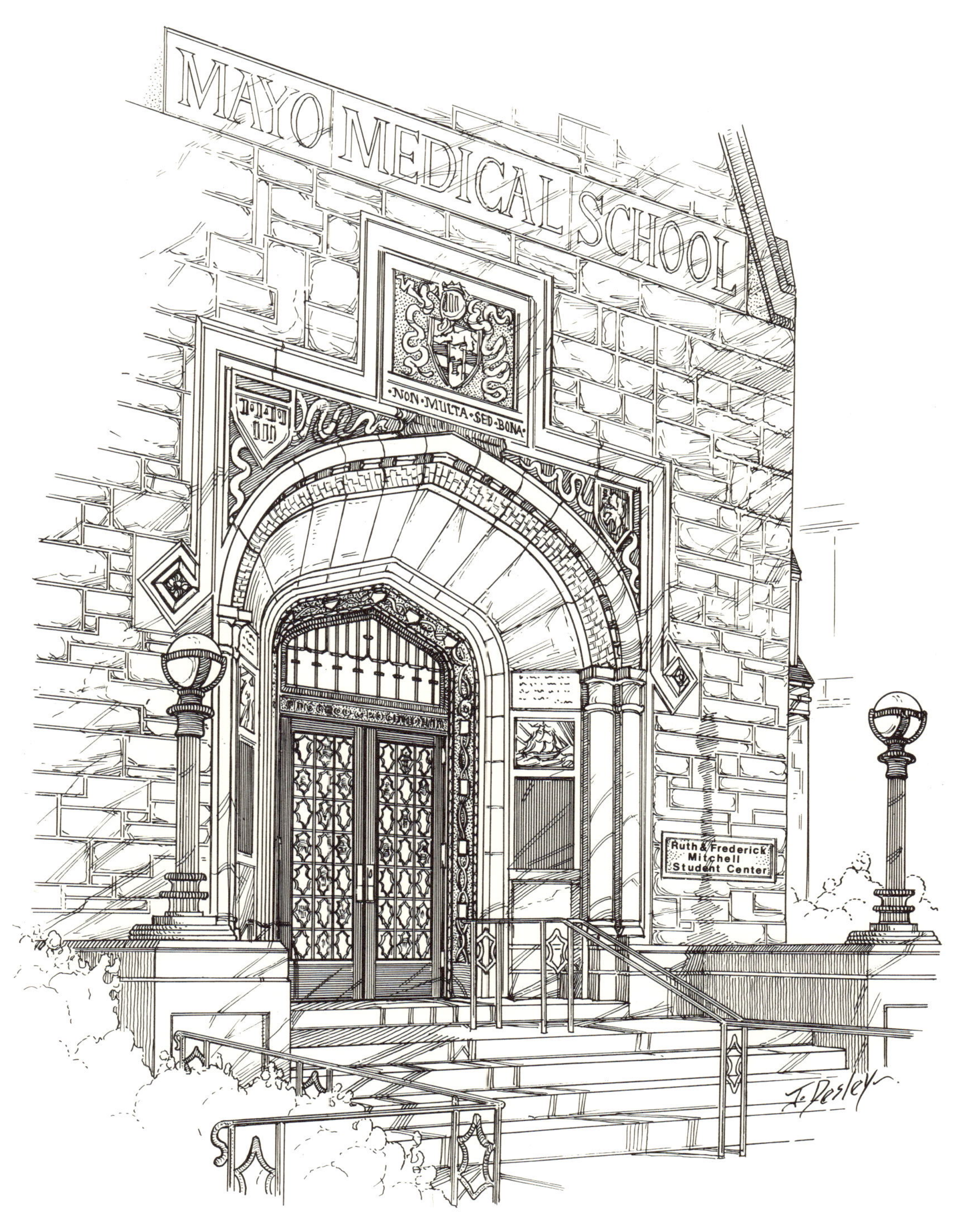
MAYO MEDICAL SCHOOL
NON MULTA SED BONA
Ruth & Frederick Mitchell Student Center

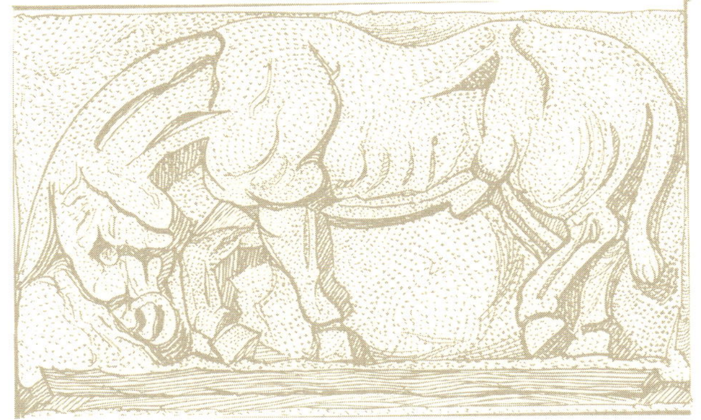

"My original drawing of the tower section didn't include the two Catholic sisters, dressed in traditional habits, ambling peacefully along in the foreground. I added them to symbolize the compassionate, caring attitudes and the consistent, persistent, dedication of the Sisters of Saint Francis to whom much credit should be given for Mayo's remarkable success."—JWD

Saint Marys Hospital *(Tower Section)*

(Plate 10)

The tower section of the Francis Building has long been a focal point of the sprawling Saint Marys Hospital campus. The building was dedicated in 1941. This view of the north facade features the ornate door that, for many years, served as the hospital's main entrance. Through the years the staff and facilities at Saint Marys have consistently provided sophisticated technical, medical, and surgical services in an atmosphere marked by Christian compassion and charity.

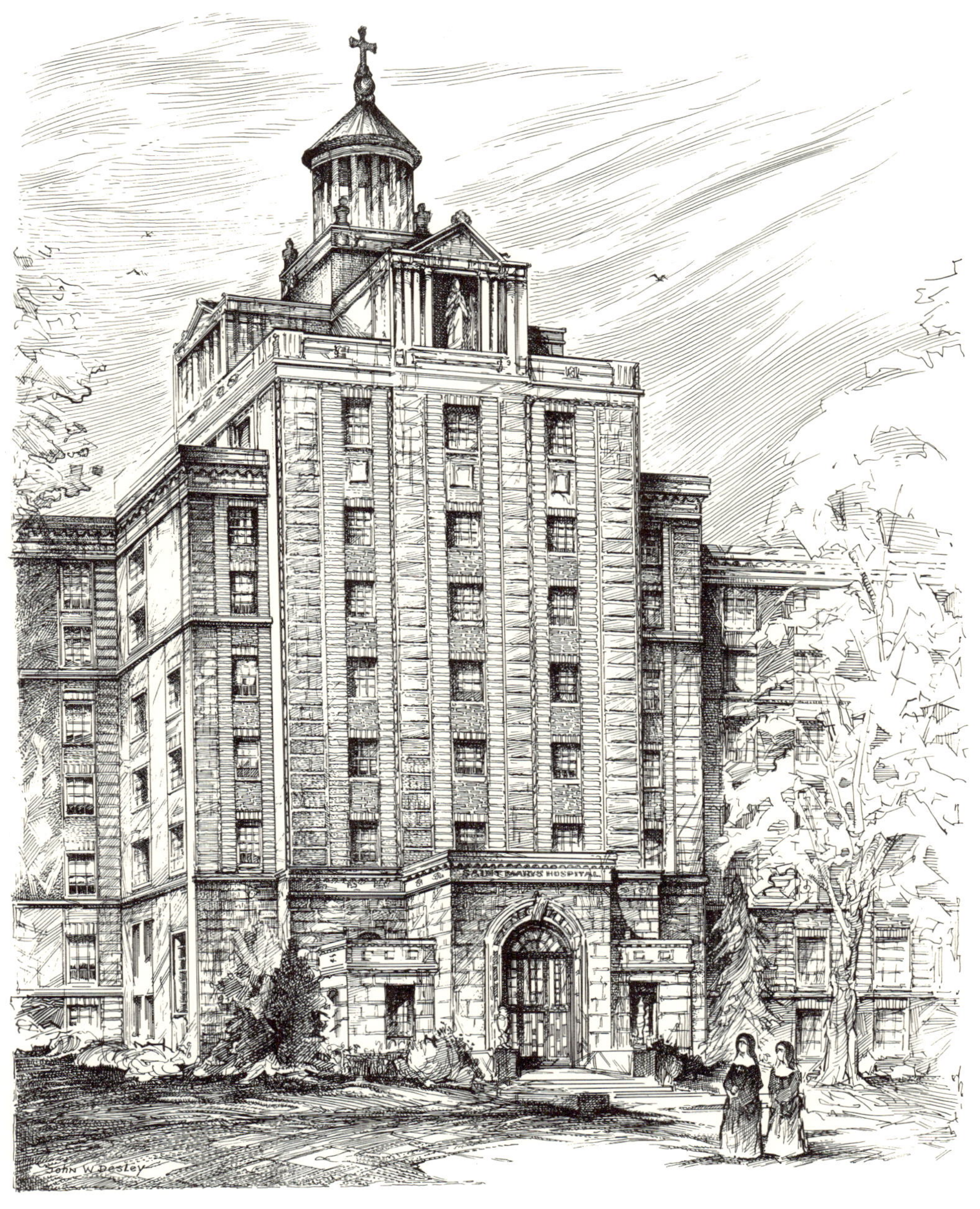
SAINT MARYS HOSPITAL

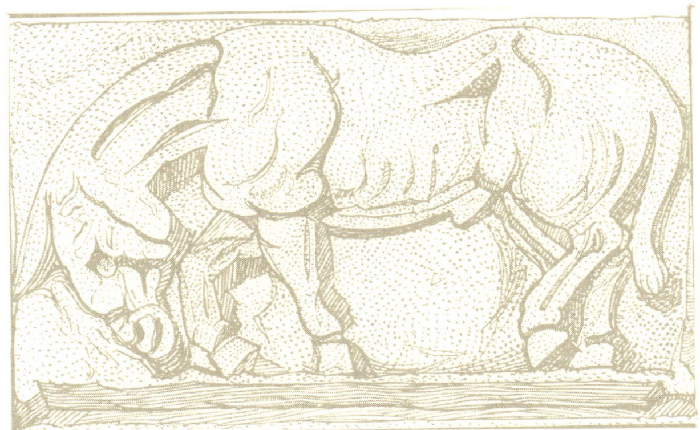

Saint Marys Hospital ***(North Facade)***

(Plate 11)

As the Mayo Clinic practice grew, so did Saint Marys Hospital. A devastating tornado in 1883 led Mother Alfred Moes, of the Sisters of Saint Francis, to champion construction of the original hospital (not shown). Four years of hard work and frugal living by the Sisters enabled them to purchase nine acres of land for $2,200. The hospital opened in 1889 with 45 beds and one operating room. Dr. William Worrall Mayo, father of Drs. William J. and Charles H. Mayo, was first director of the medical staff. Under the sponsorship of the Sisters of Saint Francis, originally a Catholic charitable teaching order, the hospital expanded over the years. This view of the north facade features the Joseph and Francis buildings.

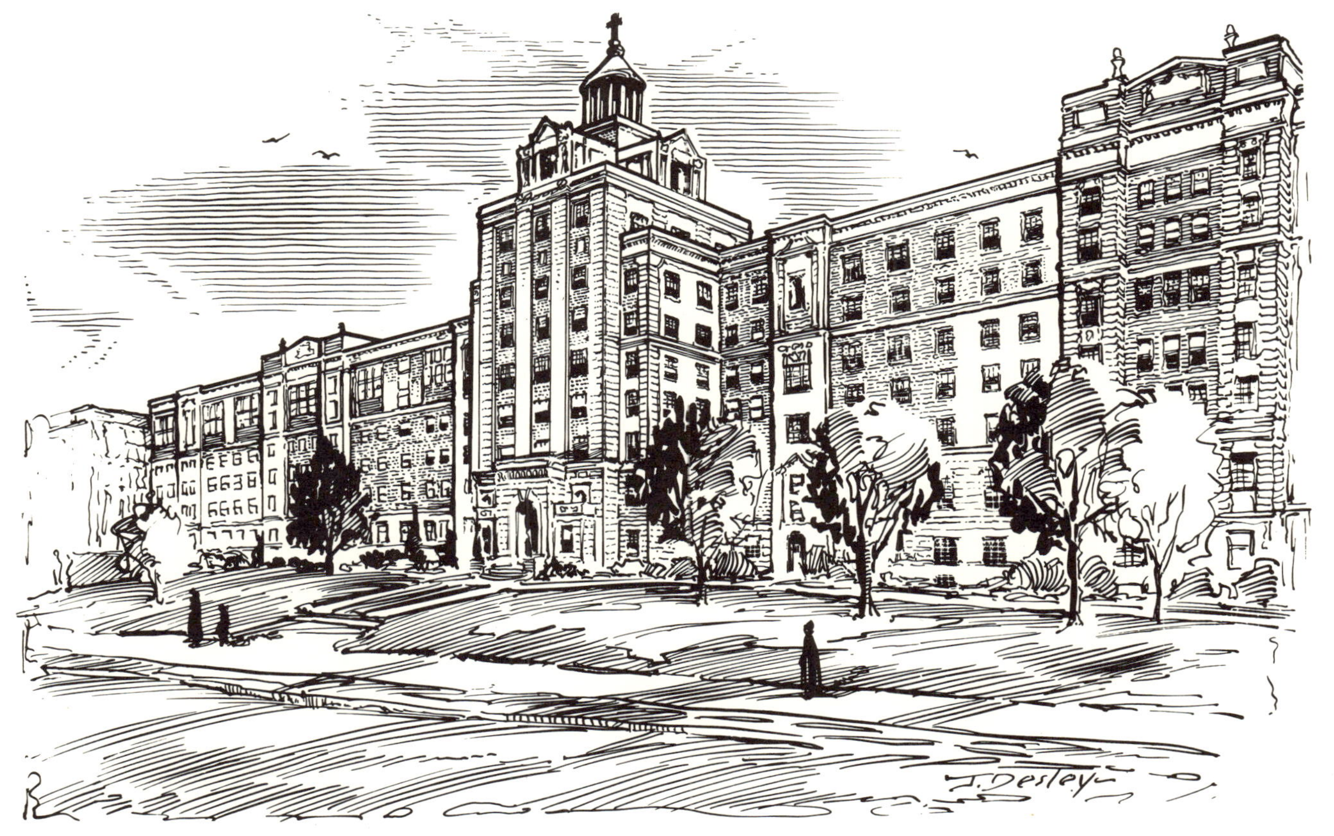
J. Desley

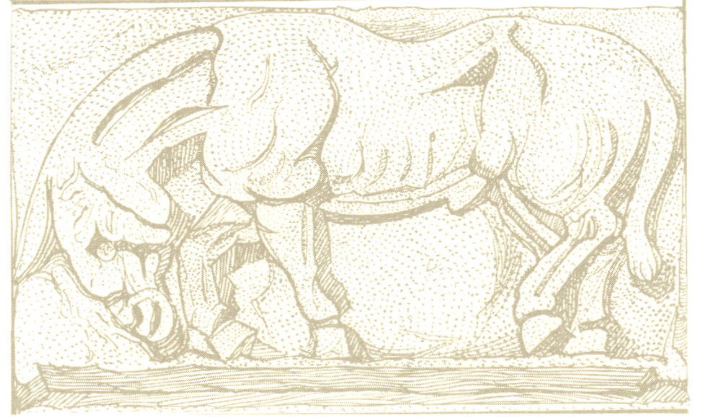

"Progress, growth, and change are integral to the Mayo tradition and culture. Even as I was finishing this drawing, yet another addition was under construction on this side of the Saint Marys Hospital complex."—JWD

Saint Marys Hospital *(West Facade)*

(Plate 12)

With more than 1,000 beds and 45 operating rooms, Saint Marys Hospital is one of the largest, best-equipped private hospitals in the world. This view depicts some of the newer additions to the hospital's west side, including the Trauma Center's rooftop helicopter landing site.

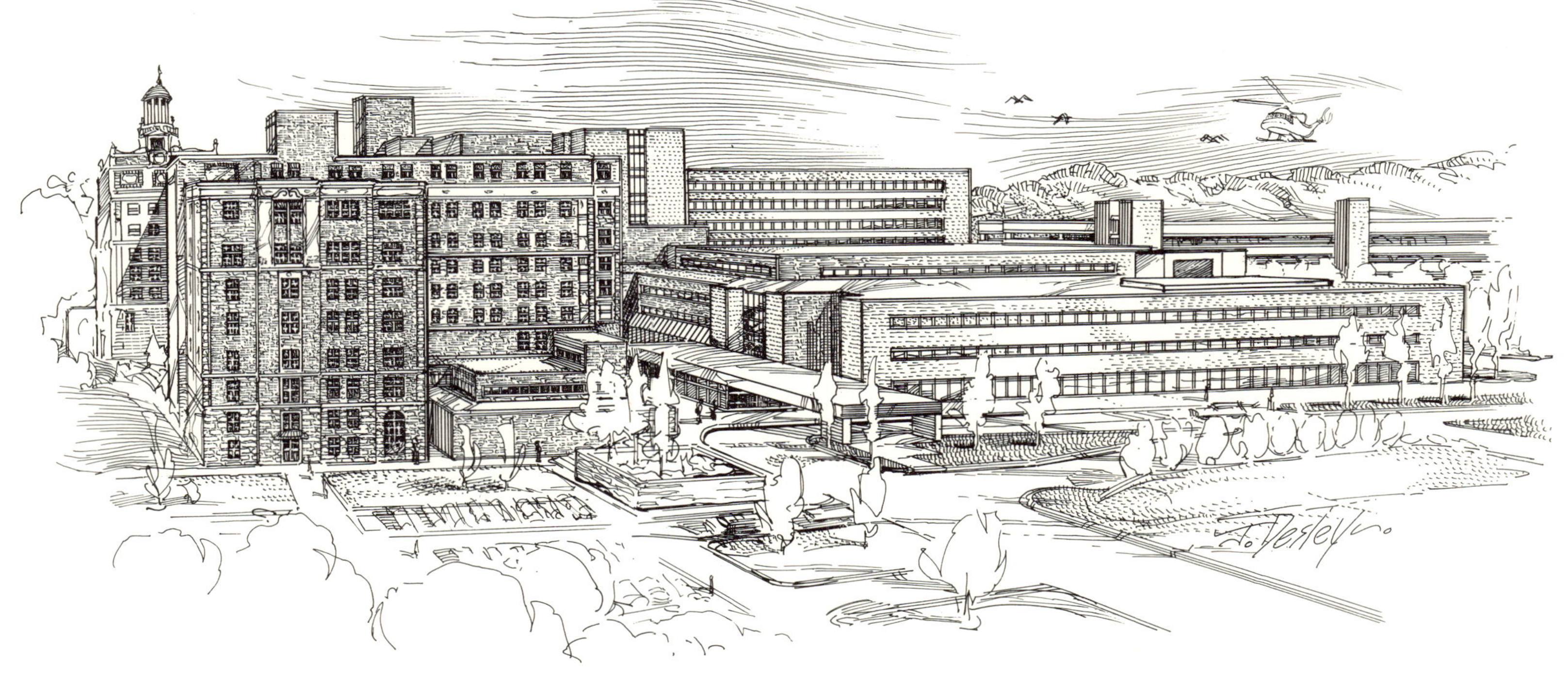

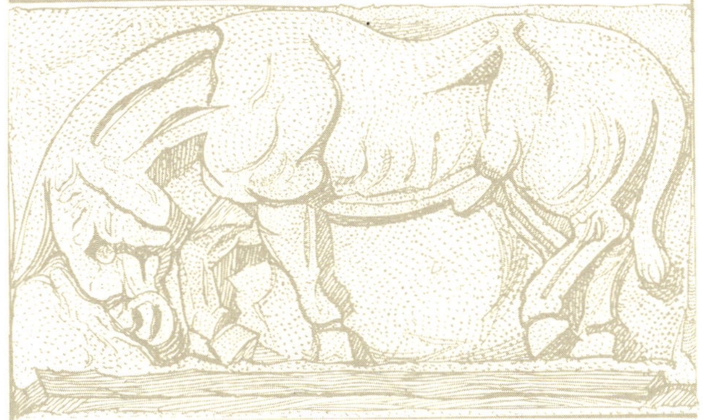

Genererose Building *(Saint Marys Hospital)*

(Plate 13)

The Generose Building, located on the southwest side of the Saint Marys Hospital campus, is a state-of-the-art psychiatry and psychology treatment center. The building was named in honor of former Saint Marys Hospital administrator Sister Generose Gervais and dedicated in 1993.

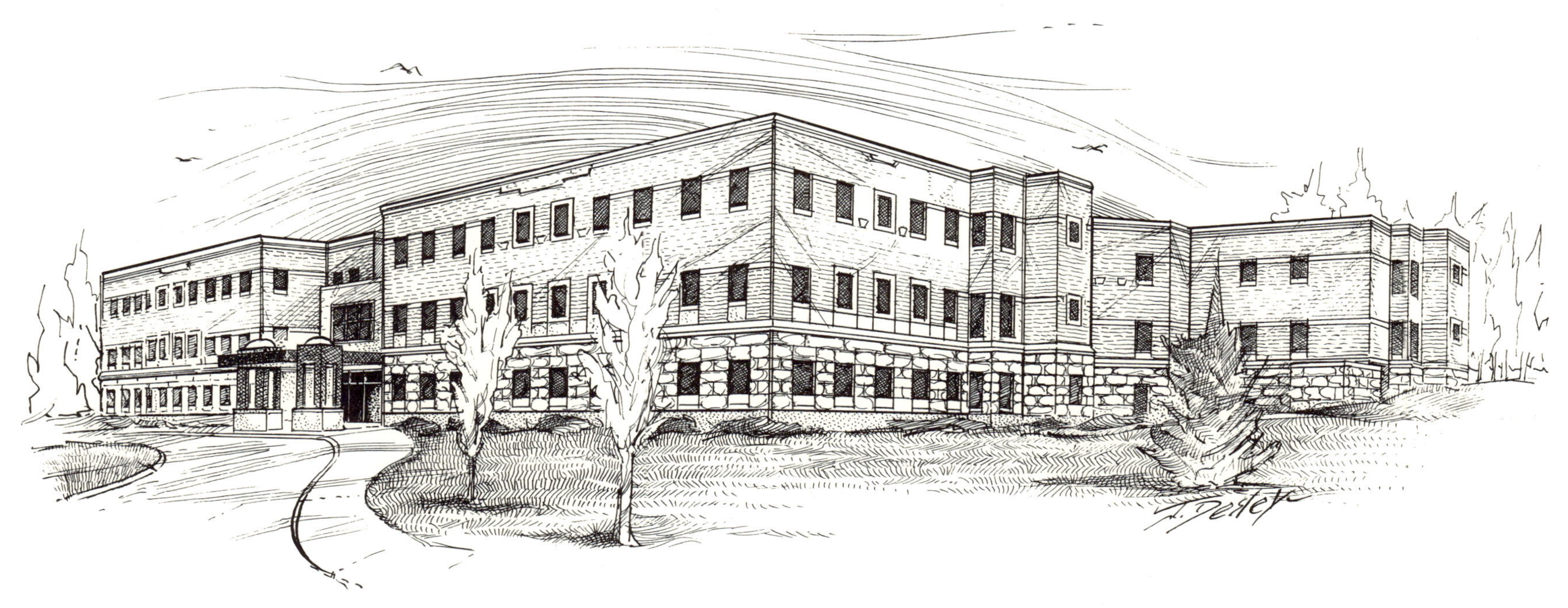

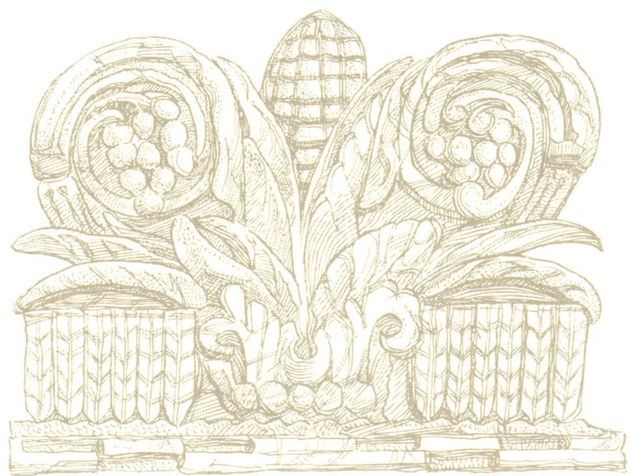

Rochester Methodist Hospital *(Southeast Facade)* *(Plate 14)*

Rochester Methodist Hospital has long played an important role in the growth and success of Mayo Medical Center. Dedication ceremonies for the hospital occurred in 1954, after the not-for-profit Methodist Hospital Corporation assumed control of the Kahler Corporation's Colonial and Worrall hospitals and properties. The modern facility was dedicated in 1966. In 1989 the hospital's main building was named in honor of Chicago industrialist George M. Eisenberg, a longtime Mayo patient and one of Mayo's principal benefactors. Today, Rochester Methodist Hospital has more than 550 beds and 34 operating rooms. This view features the southeast corner of the hospital.

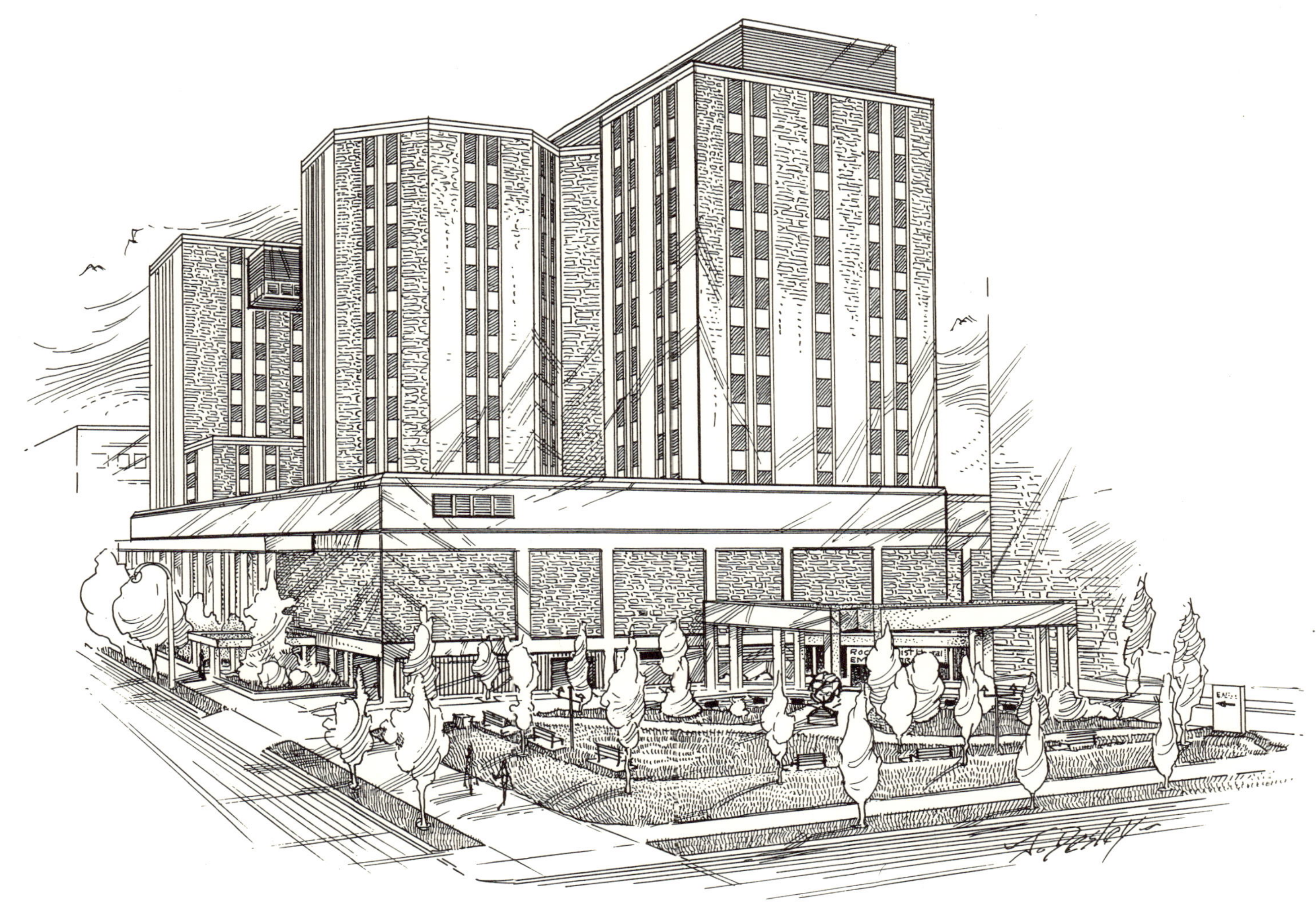

(Plate 14)

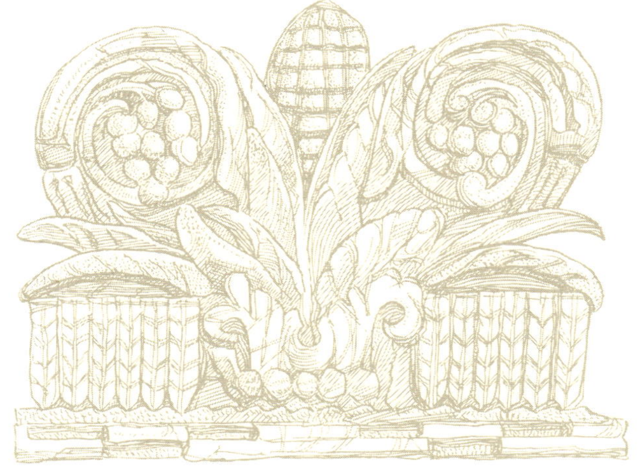

"Administrators at Rochester Methodist Hospital asked me to create this drawing for use in a hospital brochure. It posed a challenge in that construction work on the Charlton Building, which was subsequently added to the hospital's west side, was underway at the time of the commissioning."—JWD

Rochester Methodist Hospital ***(Southwest Facade)***

(Plate 15)

This view of Rochester Methodist Hospital features an attractive west-side addition completed in 1977.

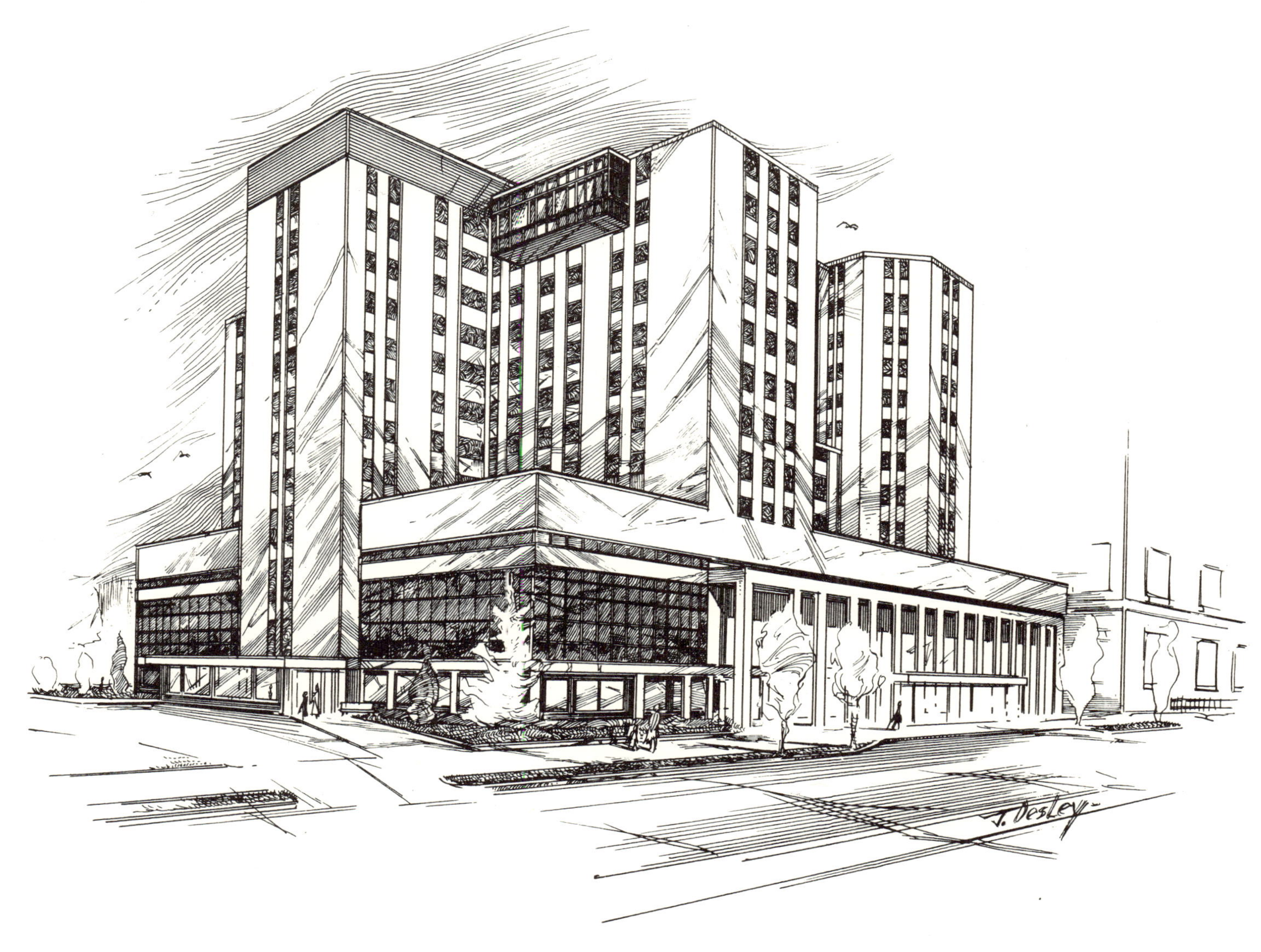

(Plate 15)

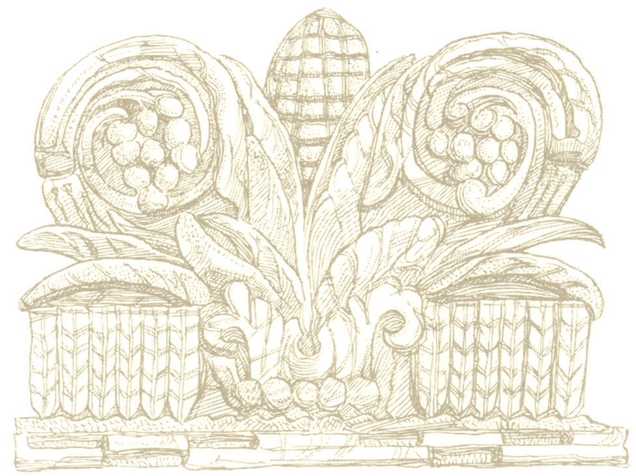

Charlton Building

(Plate 16)

The Charlton Building, attached directly to Rochester Methodist Hospital, was dedicated in 1989. It is designed and equipped to provide a wide variety of care and support services for patients in the hospital as well as Mayo Clinic outpatients. A heliport on the rooftop makes the hospital accessible to Mayo's air ambulance service. The six-story building was named in honor of the Charlton family of Fall River and Westport Harbor, Massachusetts, and in recognition of the philanthropy of Ruth Charlton Mitchell Masson.

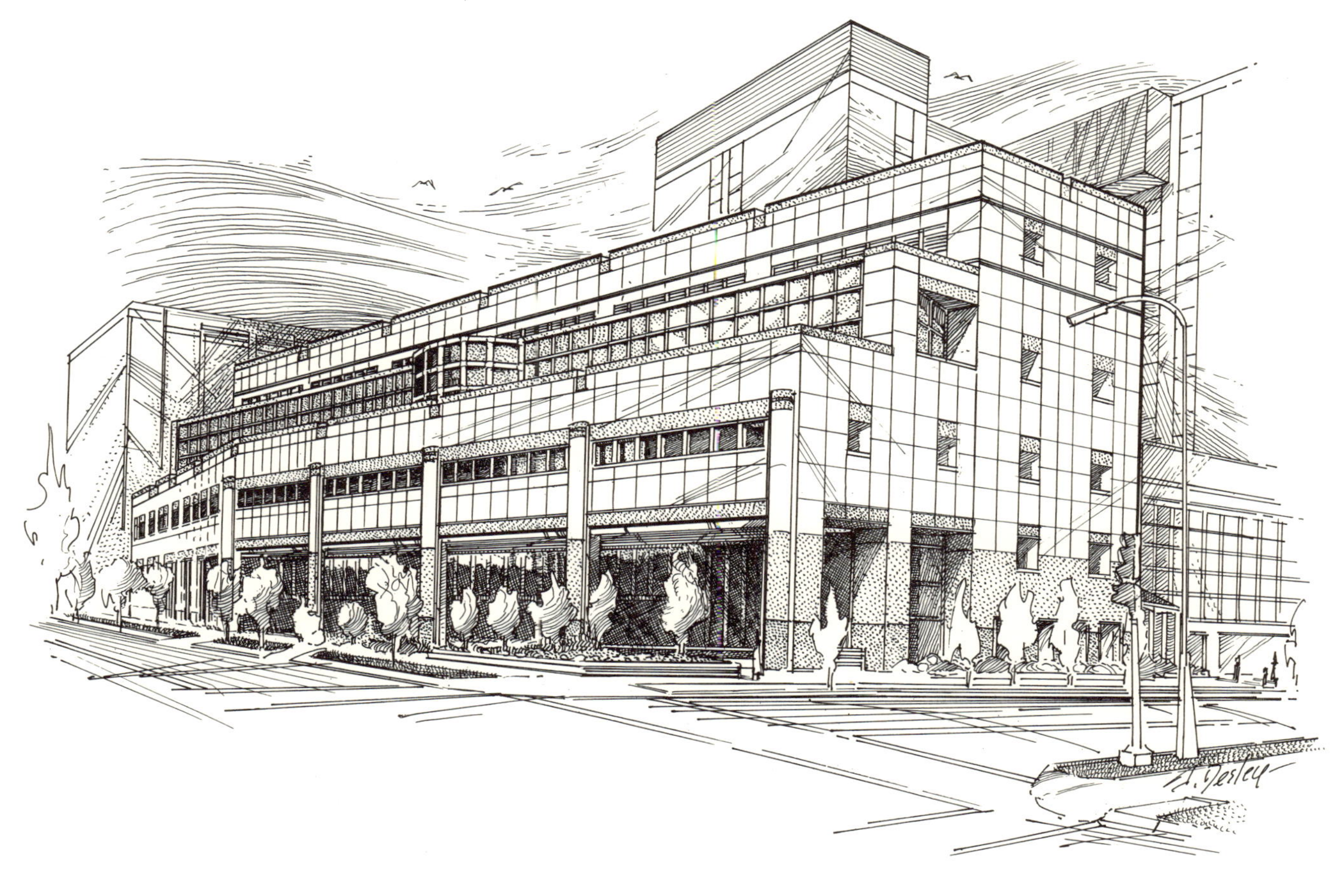

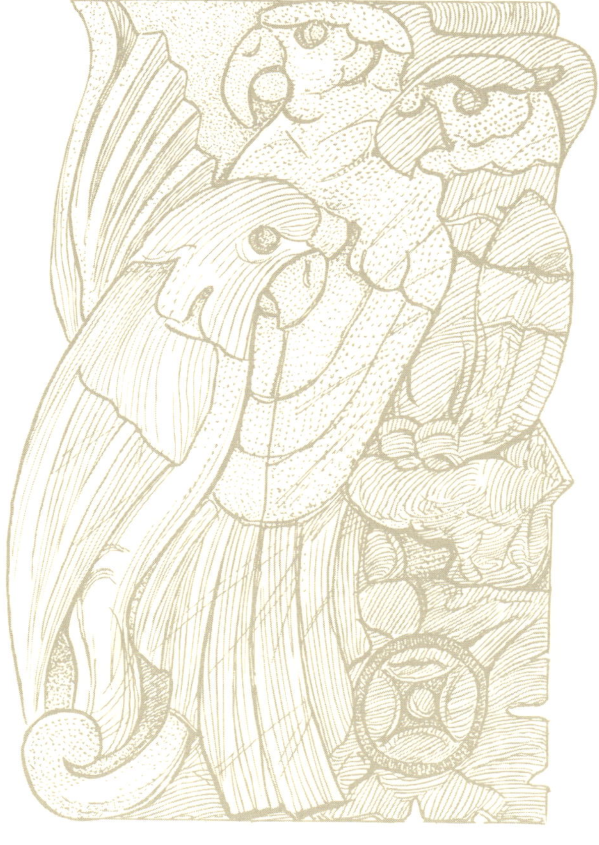

Hilton and Guggenheim Buildings

(Plate 17)

The Conrad N. Hilton Building for Laboratory Medicine, left, was made possible by a gift from the late Conrad N. Hilton. The Murry and Leonie Guggenheim Building for Research and Education in the Life Sciences, right, was funded, in part, by a gift from the Murry and Leonie Guggenheim Foundation. Nestled between the taller buildings is the Mitchell Student Center, Mayo Medical School. The Hilton and Guggenheim buildings were originally constructed in the mid 1970s. Additional floors were added to accommodate expansions in Mayo laboratory medicine and research programs (see page 39).

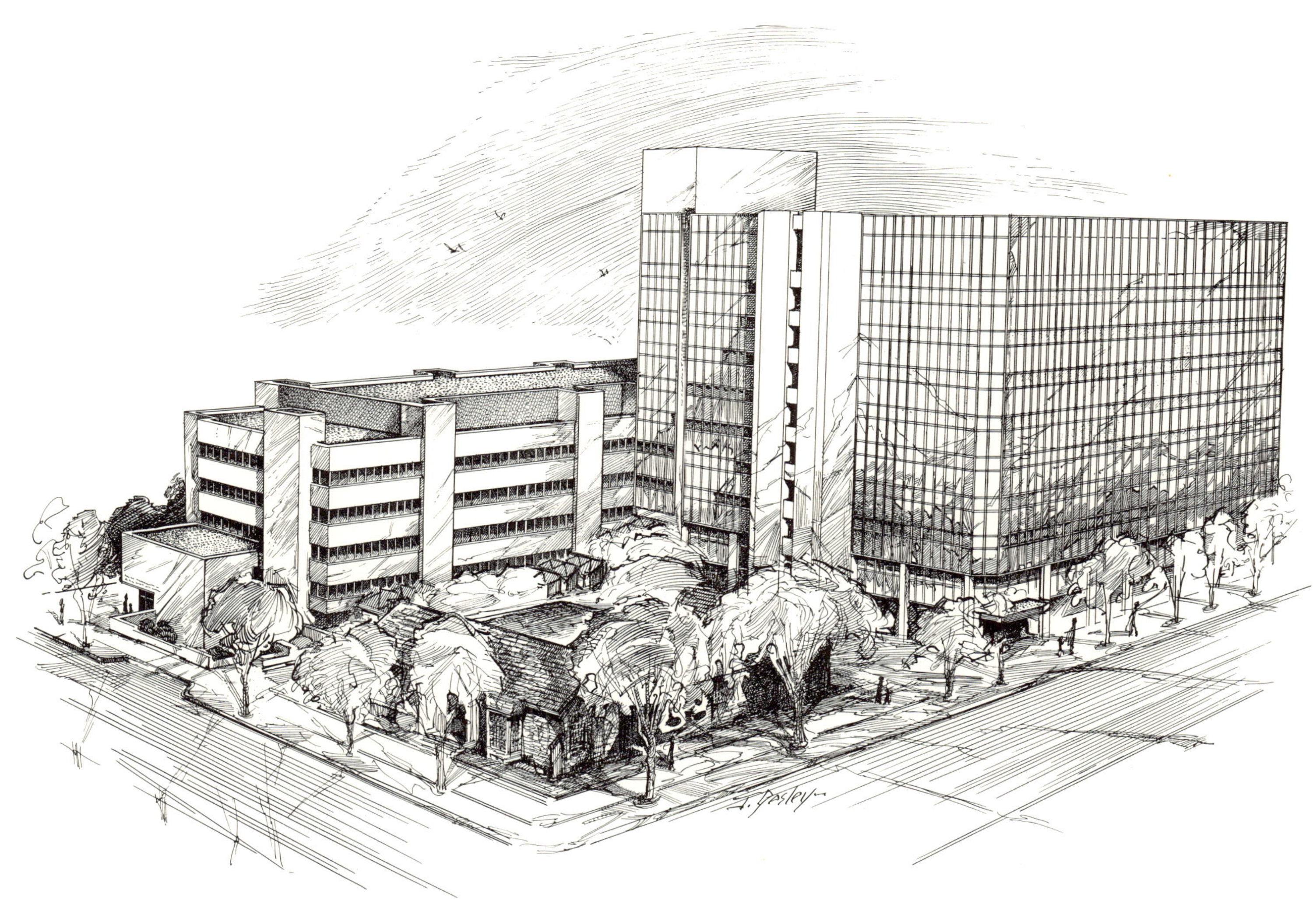

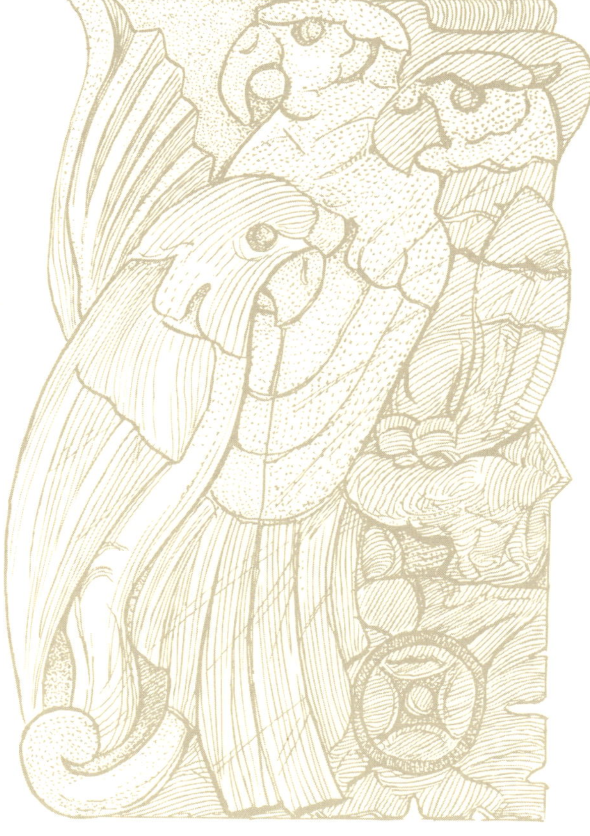

Hilton and Guggenheim Buildings

(Plate 18)

The expanded Hilton and Guggenheim buildings as they appear today. Foreground: Mitchell Student Center, Mayo Medical School.

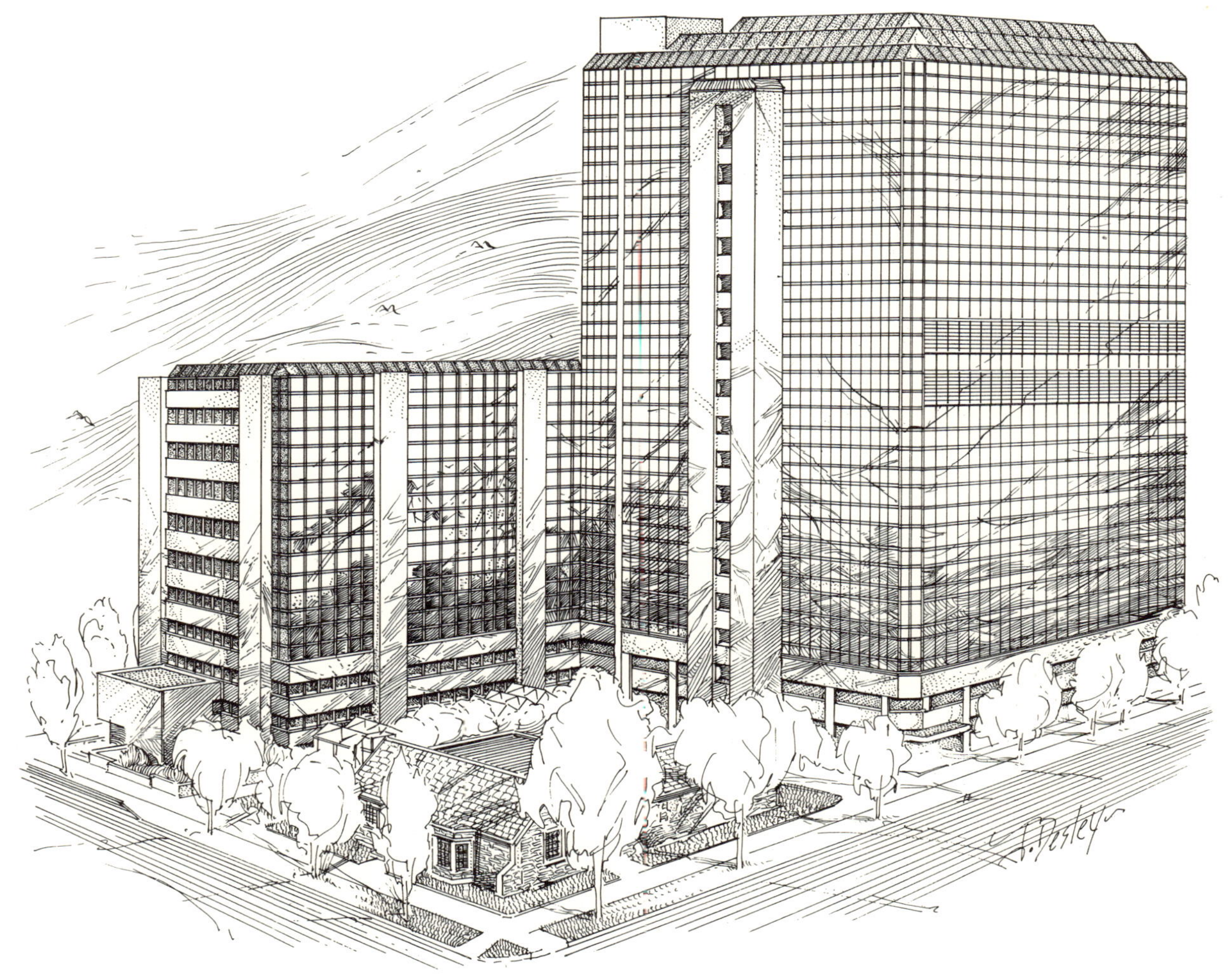

(Plate 18)

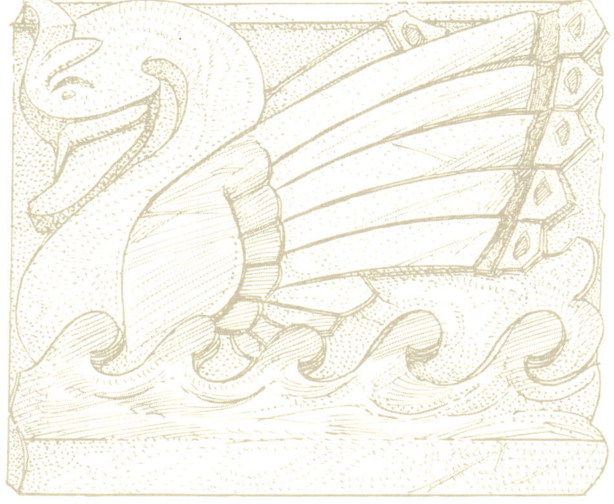

"The Siebens Building architects did a wonderful job in designing a contemporary structure that blends so well with a landmark. Before beginning this drawing I hadn't noticed just how closely the beautiful new and old buildings resemble one another."—JWD

Siebens and Plummer Buildings

(Plate 19)

The Harold W. Siebens Medical Education Building, left, opened in 1989. It was named in honor of the benefactor whose philanthropy and challenge enabled this to be the first building at Mayo funded entirely by private contributions. The building is linked to the Plummer Building, right, which was completed in 1928. The Siebens Building stands on a two-time historic site. This was the location of Dr. and Mrs. William Worrall Mayo's home, which was removed to make room for construction of the 1914 Mayo Clinic Building (see page 55).

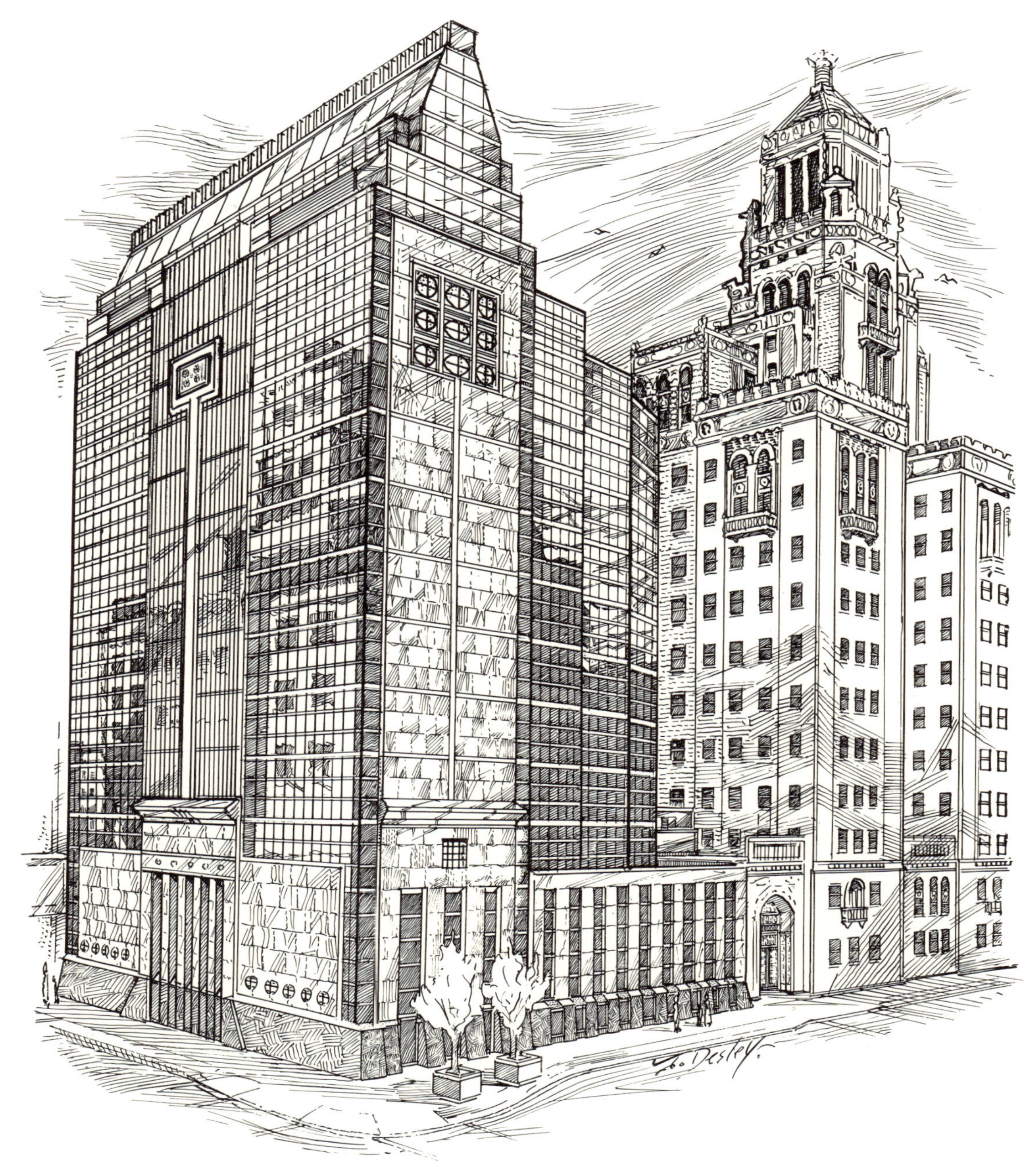

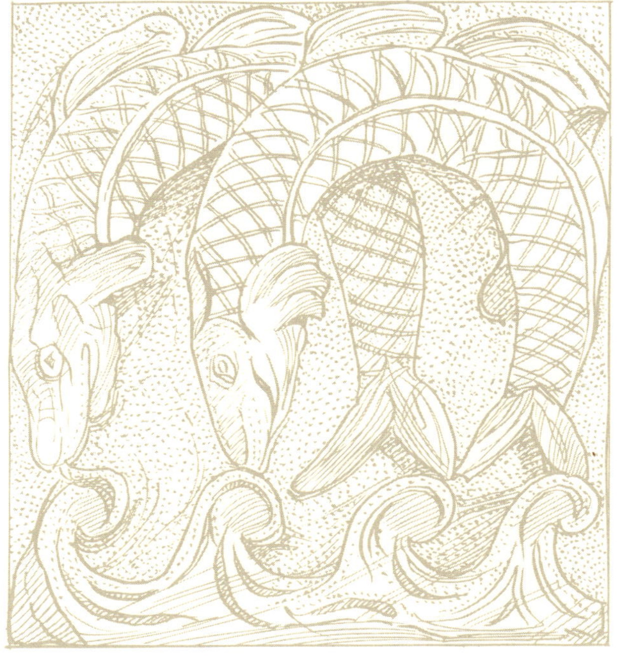

"Doctor and Mrs. William J. Mayo designed their home to be an extension of the Mayo clinical facilities, often hosting parties for visiting medical and political dignitaries, sometimes putting them up overnight. Balfour Hall is an elegant, spacious, third-floor room that was used for entertaining, mainly dancing."—JWD

Mayo Foundation House

(Plate 20)

Mayo Foundation House is the spacious former home of Dr. and Mrs. William J. Mayo. The home has 47 rooms and a five-story tower like the one in which Dr. Mayo, as a child, observed his mother as she pursued her hobby of astronomy. The home has an elevator and a pipe organ. Its design is reminiscent of an English manor house. In 1938, Dr. and Mrs. Mayo contributed their home to Mayo Foundation for use as a meeting place for the exchange of ideas "for the good of mankind." It remains a popular site for Mayo scientific, administrative, and social gatherings.

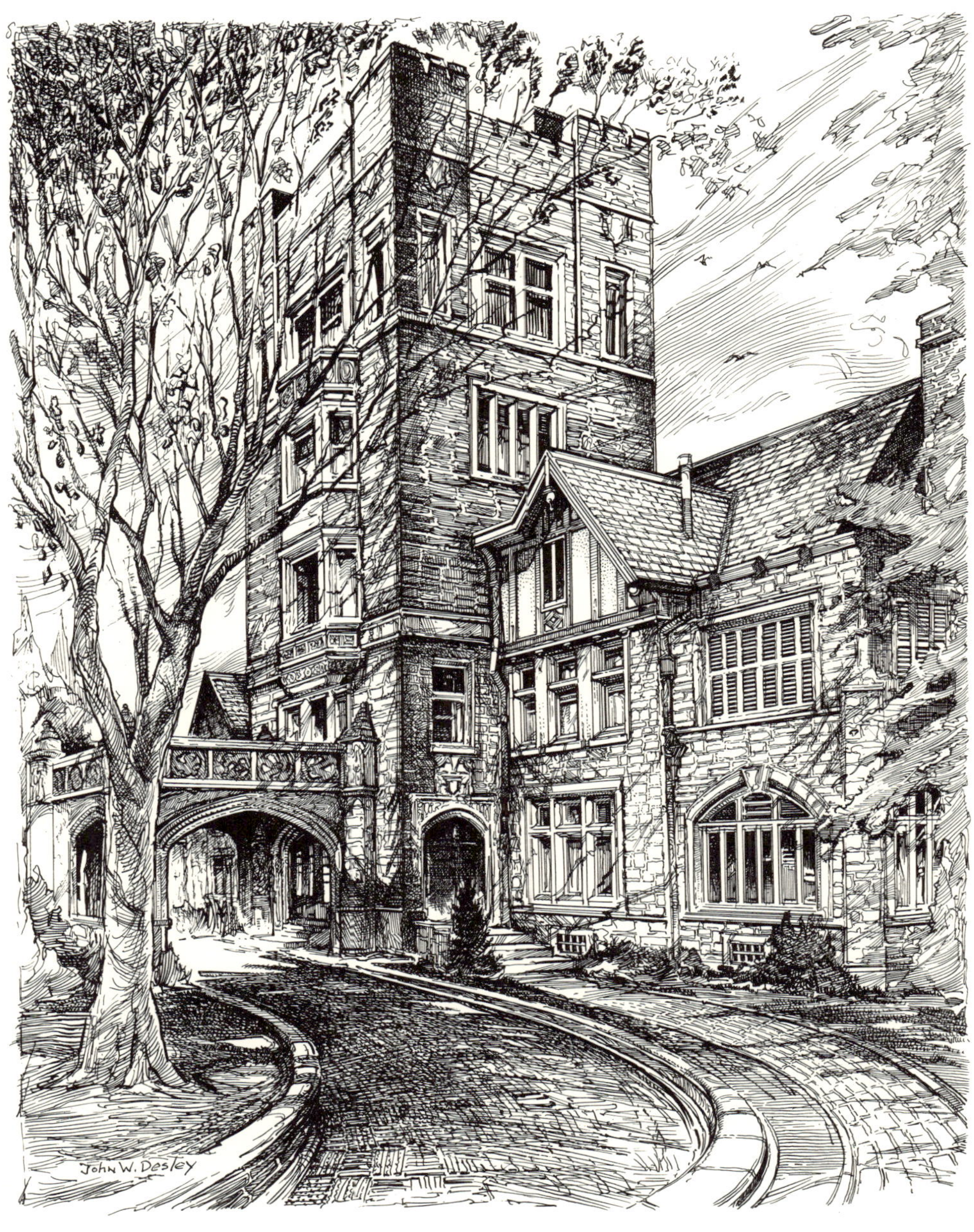

(Plate 20)

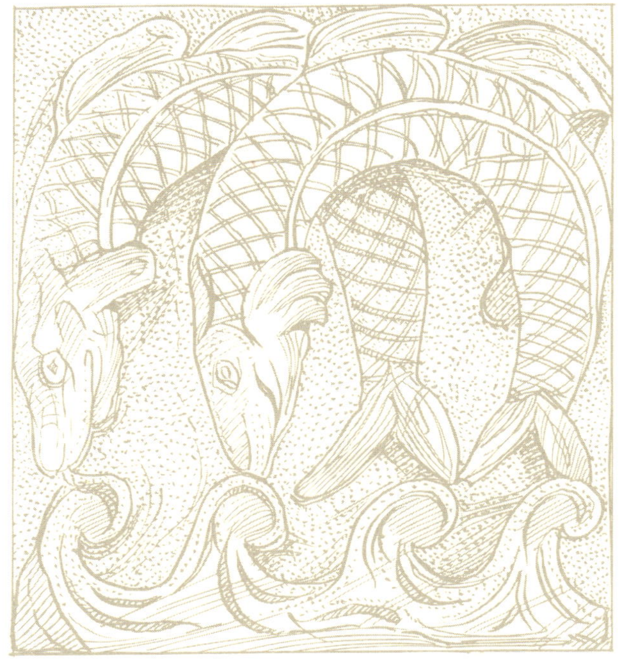

"Mayowood poses a special challenge to artists and photographers because the terrain in front of the huge home slopes away and doesn't offer a good vantage point. I wanted to draw the house at eye level, so I climbed a tree with camera in hand to capture this perspective, on which the drawing is based."—JWD

Mayowood

(Plate 21)

Built in 1910 and 1911, the Mayowood "Big House" is the former home of Dr. and Mrs. Charles H. Mayo. Dr. Charlie, the younger of the Mayo brothers, was an avid conservationist and agriculturalist. His 3,000-acre estate was a game refuge for American and Japanese deer and other wildlife, including Canadian geese whose descendants still frequent Rochester. The Mayowood greenhouse contained many species of flowers, including more than 165 varieties of chrysanthemums. The estate included a model dairy farm noted for production of clean, pure milk. Mayowood is now owned by the Olmsted County Historical Society and is open to the public through tours.

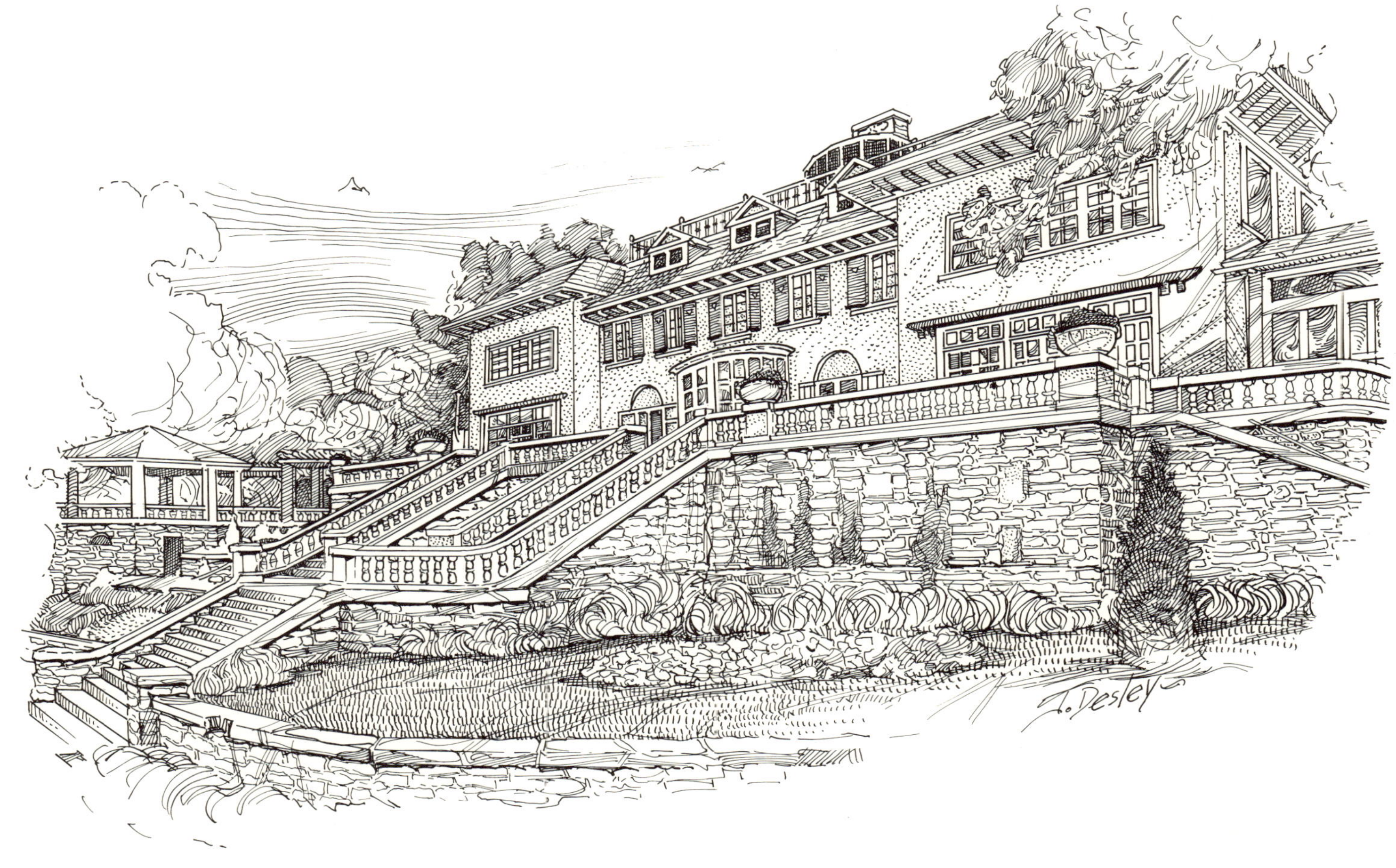

J. Desley

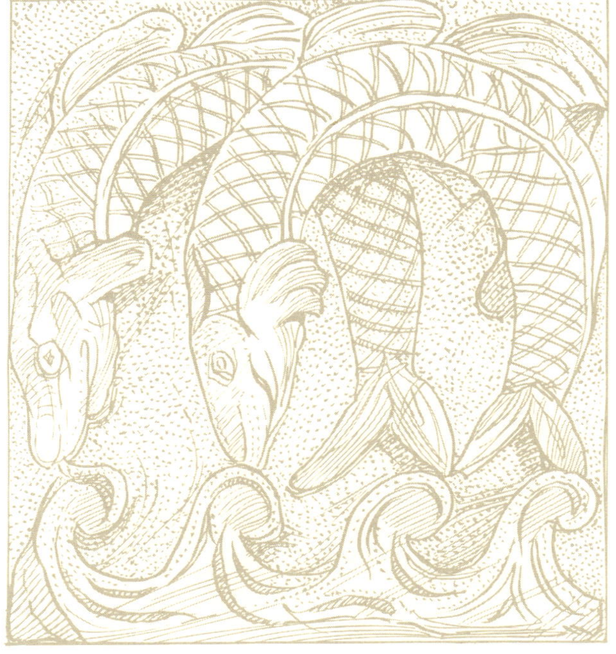

Plummer House

(Plate 22)

Dr. Henry S. Plummer began construction of his English Tudor style home in 1917 and completed it in 1924. As he later did for the Plummer Building, he personally supervised construction and formulated many innovations in the house. Plummer House, including 11 acres of beautiful grounds, gardens, trails, and a water tower, was deeded to the Rochester Art Center in 1971. It is administered by the City of Rochester Park & Recreation Department for use by people in the Rochester community.

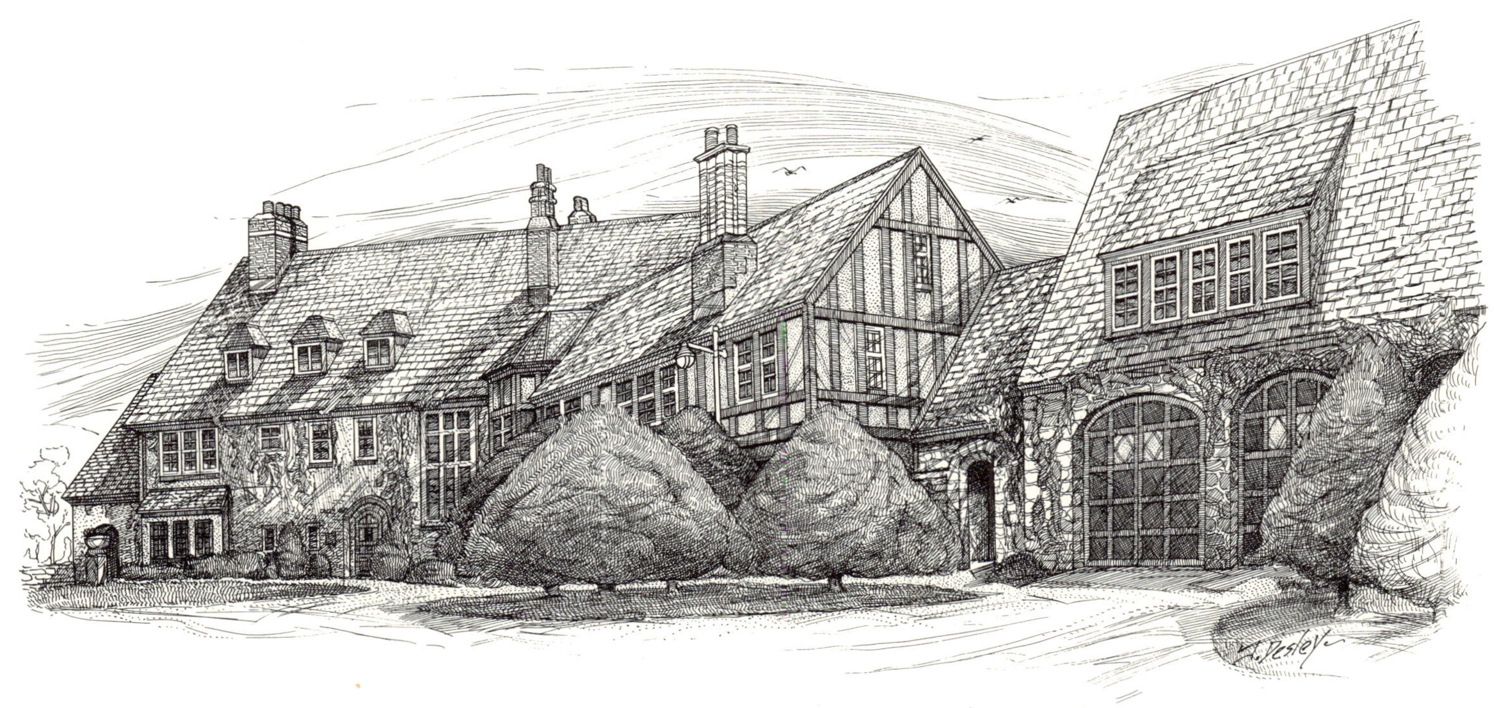

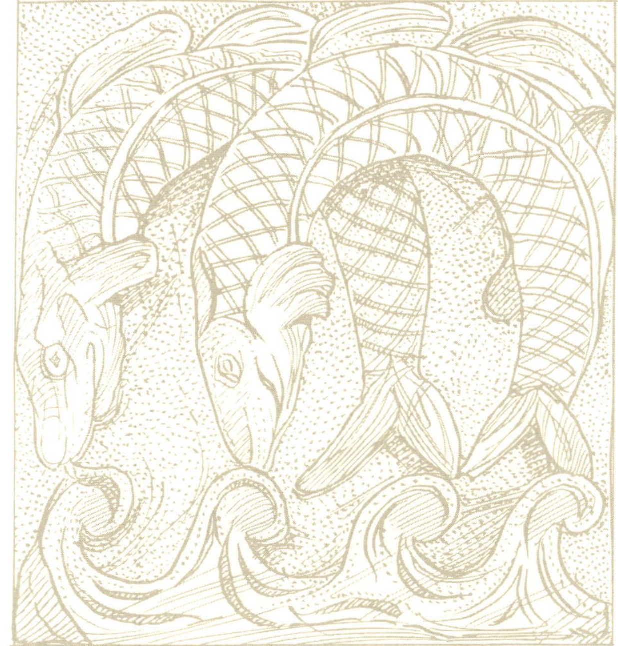

Balfour House

(Plate 23)

The Balfour country home southwest of Rochester was situated on land on which Dr. Donald Church Balfour, an internationally known Mayo surgeon and medical educator, indulged his passion for raising Holstein dairy cattle. The last partner to join the Mayo practice, his distinguished Mayo career spanned 40 years. Dr. Balfour was an original member of the Mayo Clinic Board of Governors.

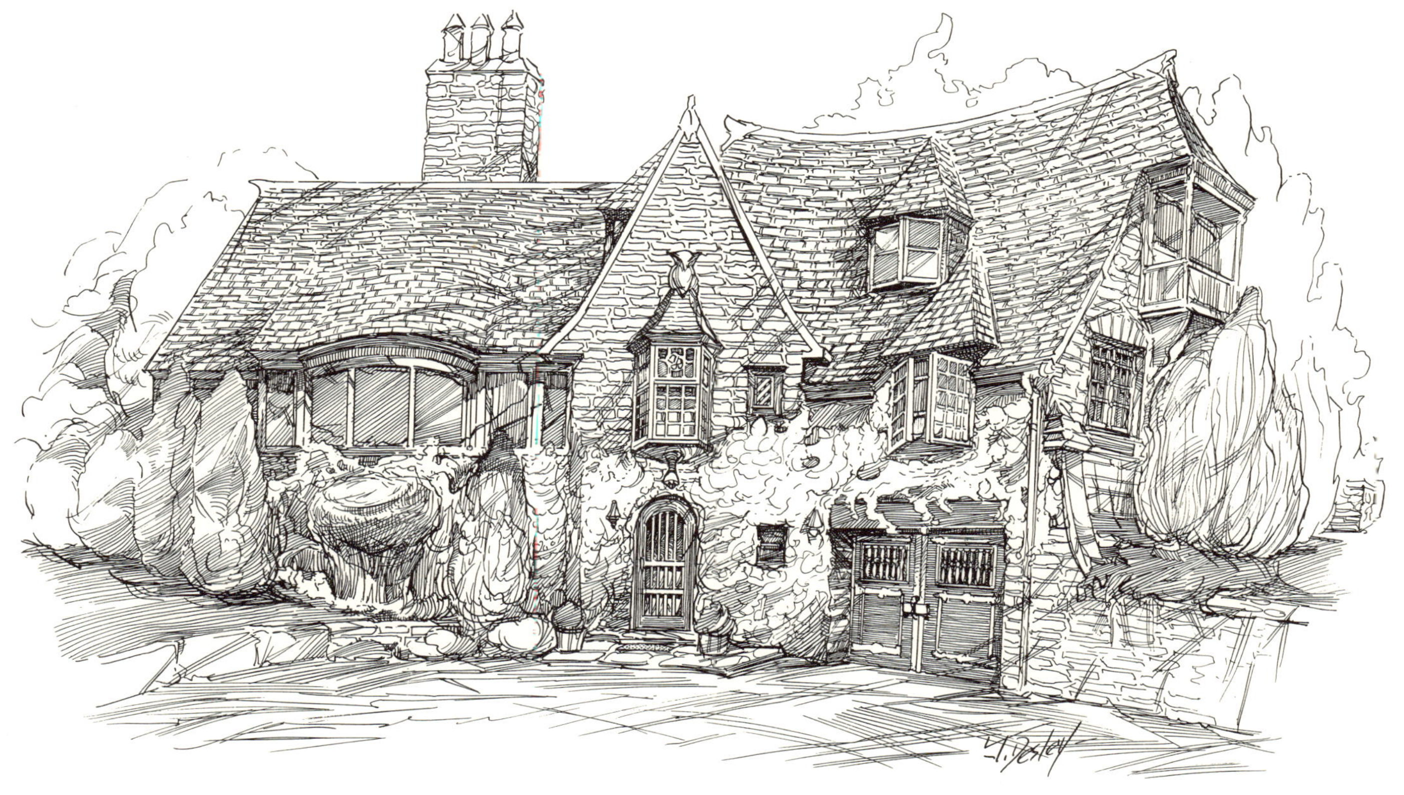

(Plate 23)

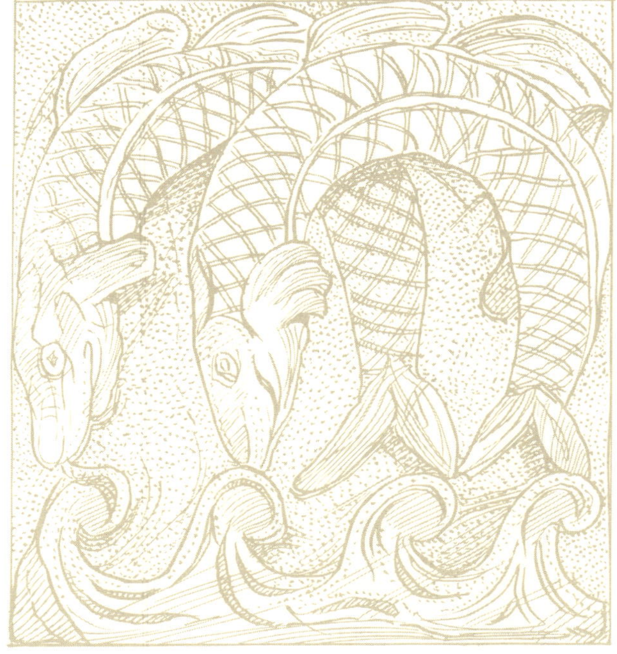

Judd House

(Plate 24)

This Georgian Colonial brick home three blocks west of the Mayo Clinic building was built for Dr. and Mrs. E. Starr Judd in 1912. Dr. Judd was a surgeon, an early partner of the Mayo brothers, and a president of the American Medical Association. The structure housed the Mayo Clinic Women's Club for more than 30 years, and then the Mayo Intensive Psychotherapy Center. Today it is home to the Gift of Life Transplant House, a facility providing high-quality, affordable accommodations in a homelike setting for Mayo patients and families of those awaiting or recovering from an organ, bone marrow or tissue transplant.

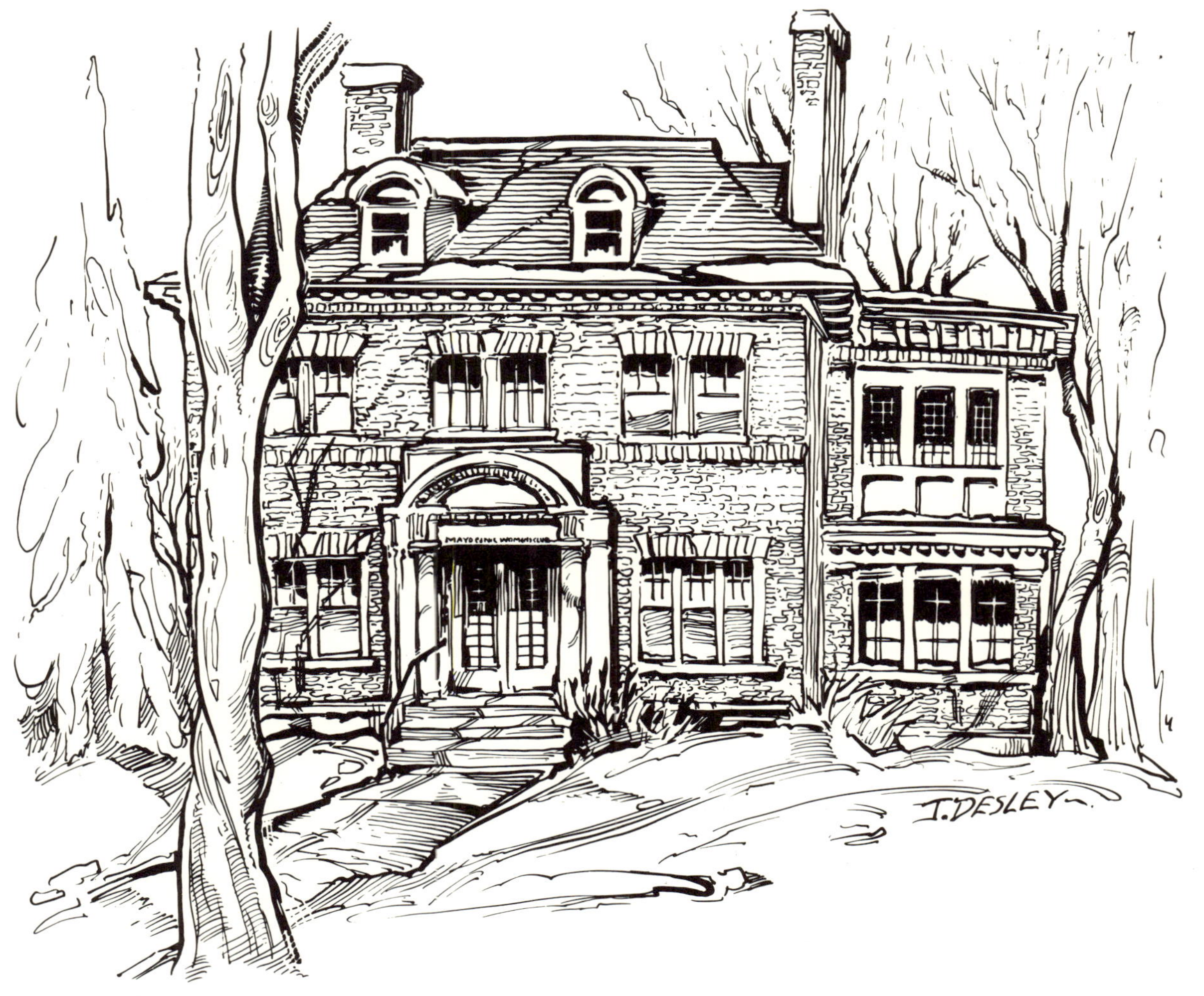
I. DESLEY

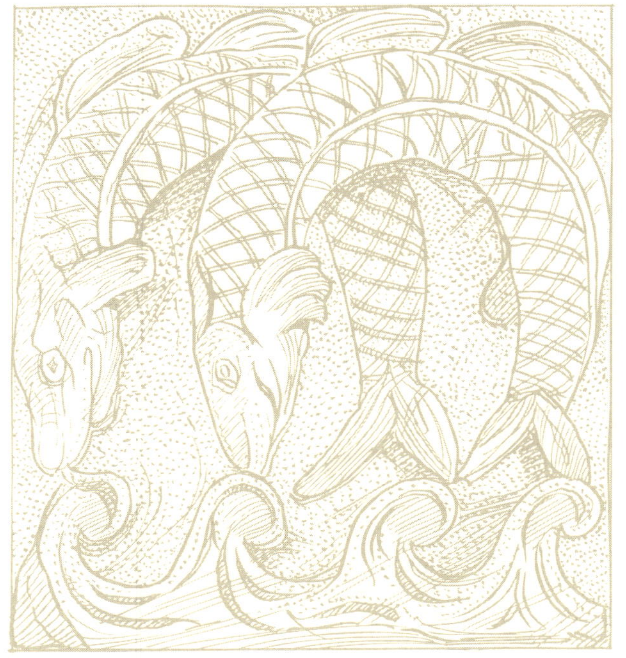

"This is a hasty sketch I made only hours before the charming residence was razed in 1973. The day started as just another day at the office, with meetings, medical illustrations, and deadlines stacking up. When I heard the news that this historic structure was to come down later that day, I packed up my pencils, walked over at noon, and captured the image for posterity."—JWD

Kahler House

(Plate 25)

Mr. and Mrs. John H. Kahler purchased this spacious southwest Rochester home in 1908 at a cost of $6,000. After investing another $1,000 in renovations, the Kahlers made it their residence. Mr. Kahler, founder and first president of the Kahler Corporation, was a close friend of Drs. William J. and Charles H. Mayo. In his seemingly fanatical loyalty to the Mayos, Mr. Kahler frequently risked his own savings to establish hotels, hospitals, laundries, and eating places required by the growing Mayo Clinic medical practice. He was appointed an honorary member of the Mayo Staff for his numerous contributions to the early Mayo practice.

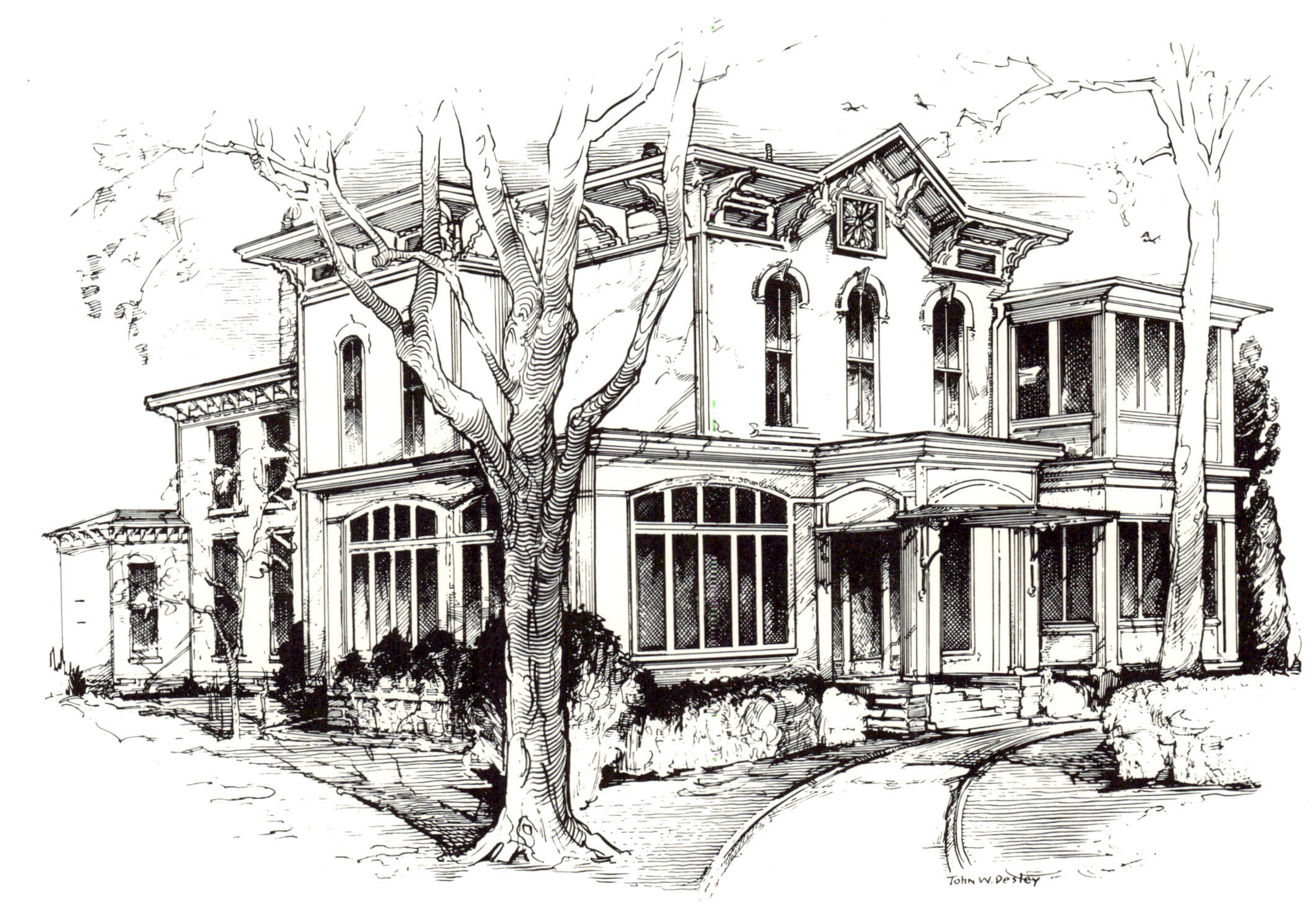
John W. Desley

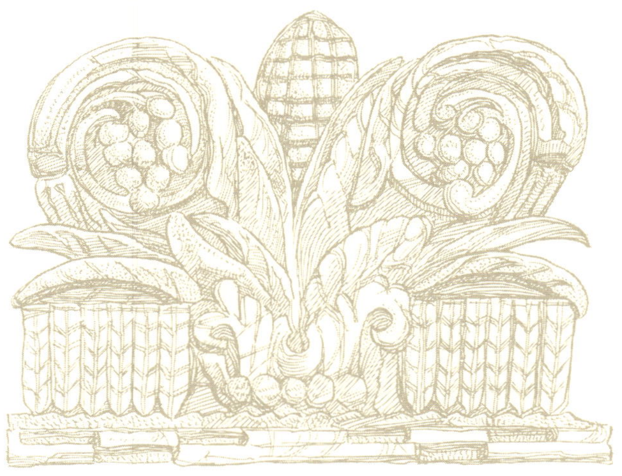

1914 Building ***(First Mayo Clinic Structure)***

(Plate 26)

The original Mayo Clinic Building, better known today as the 1914 Building, allowed the Mayos and their early associates to consolidate an integrated, coordinated, group practice in a single structure. In a cornerstone dedication ceremony in 1912, Dr. William J. Mayo stated: "The object of this building is to furnish a permanent house wherein scientific investigation can be made into the cause of the diseases which afflict mankind, and wherein every effort shall be made to cure the sick and the suffering. It is the hope of the founders of this building that in its use, the high ideals of the medical profession will always be maintained. Within its walls all classes of people, the poor as well as the rich, without regard to color or creed, shall be cared for without discrimination." The structure was razed in the 1980s to make way for the Siebens Building. In designing the new building, architects included some of the interior and exterior features of the old building.

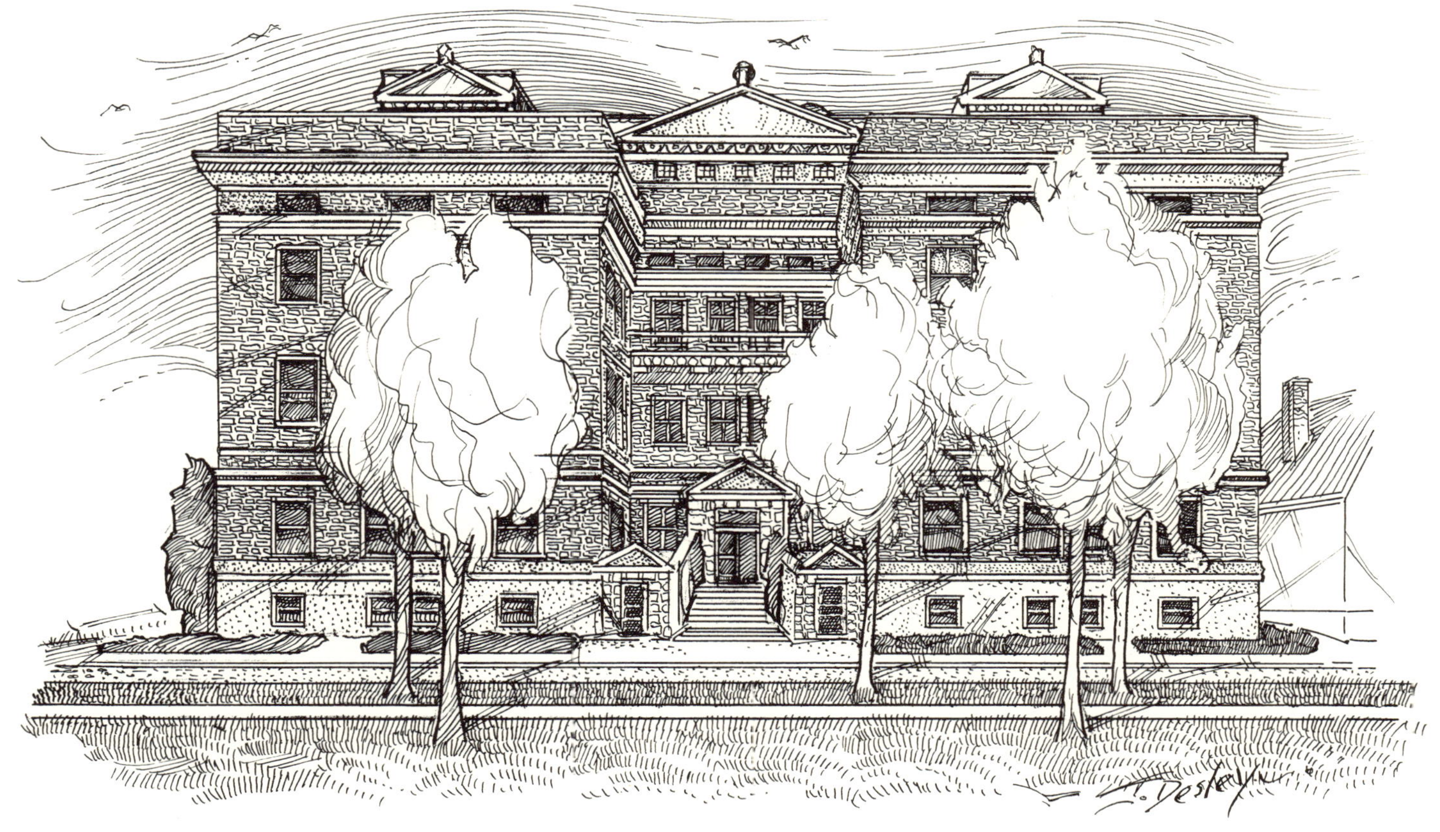

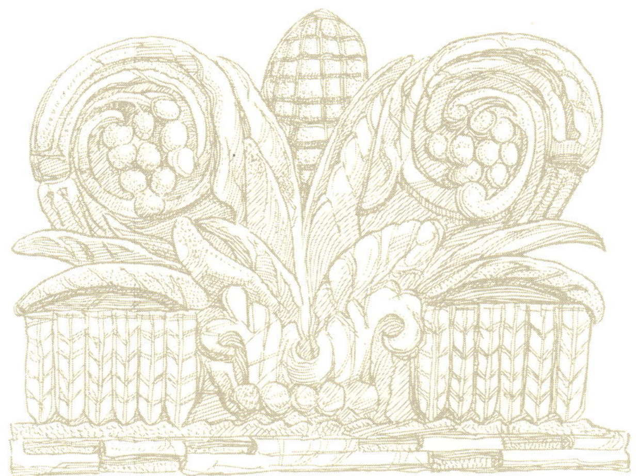

Colonial Hospital

(Plate 27)

Colonial Hospital was a forerunner of Rochester Methodist Hospital. It opened in 1915 as a hotel-hospital, blending hotel rooms with 175 hospital beds and two operating rooms for minor procedures or emergencies. Shortly thereafter the hotel rooms were abolished because of a growing need for hospital rooms. A portion of the structure remains as part of Rochester Methodist Hospital's east-side complex.

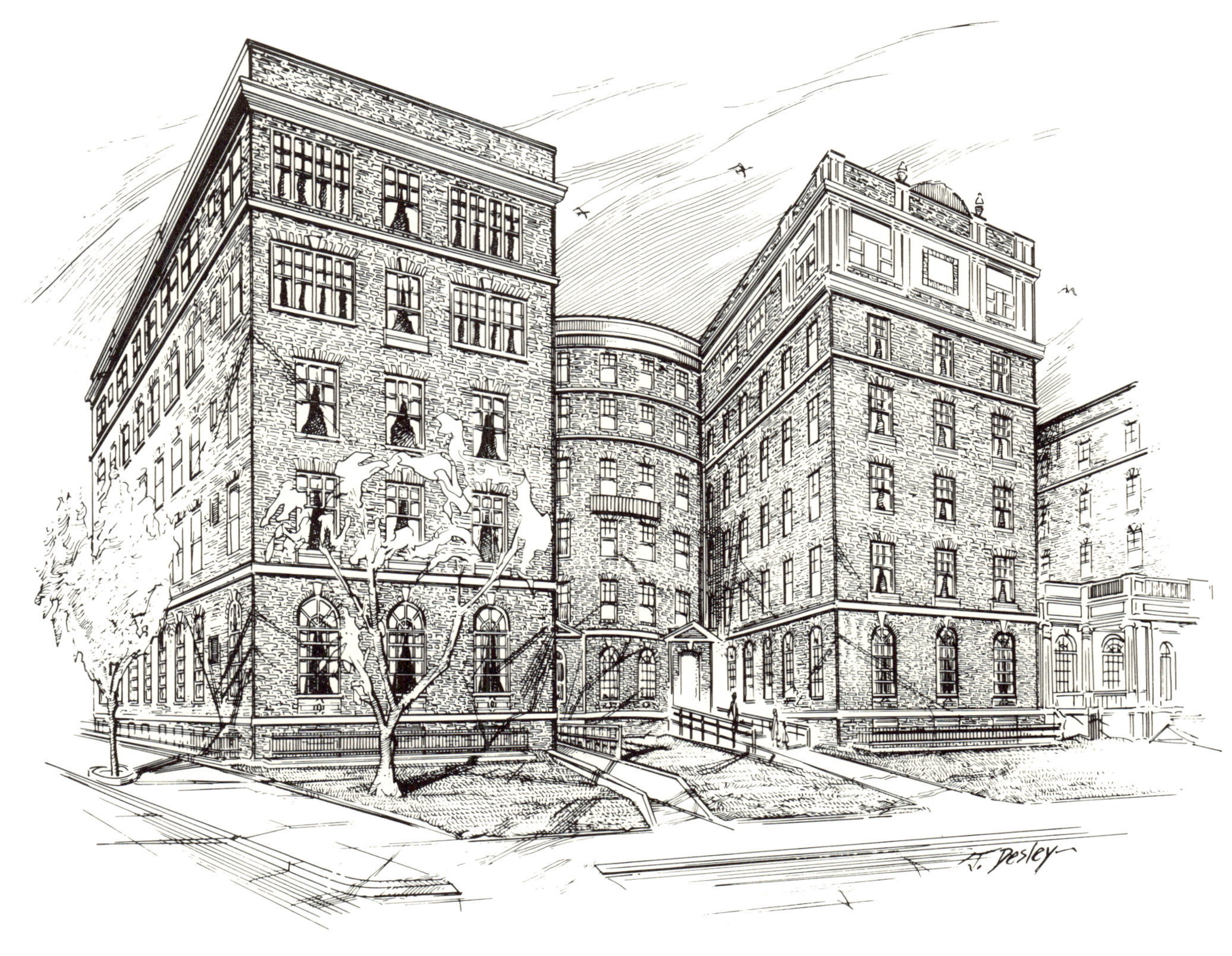

(Plate 27)

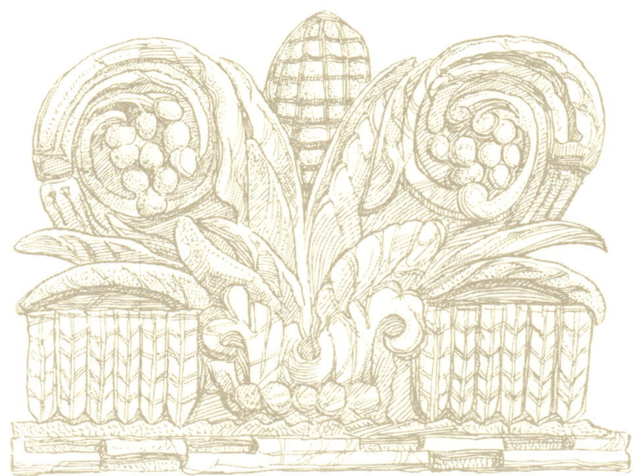

Worrall Hospital

(Plate 28)

The Worrall Hospital had an original capacity of 139 beds and included operating rooms for ophthalmology, otolaryngology, rhinology, and dentistry. This Kahler Corporation facility opened in 1919 and was named in honor of Dr. William Worrall Mayo. Later, it became part of Rochester Methodist Hospital. The structure stood on land now occupied by the Hilton and Guggenheim Buildings.

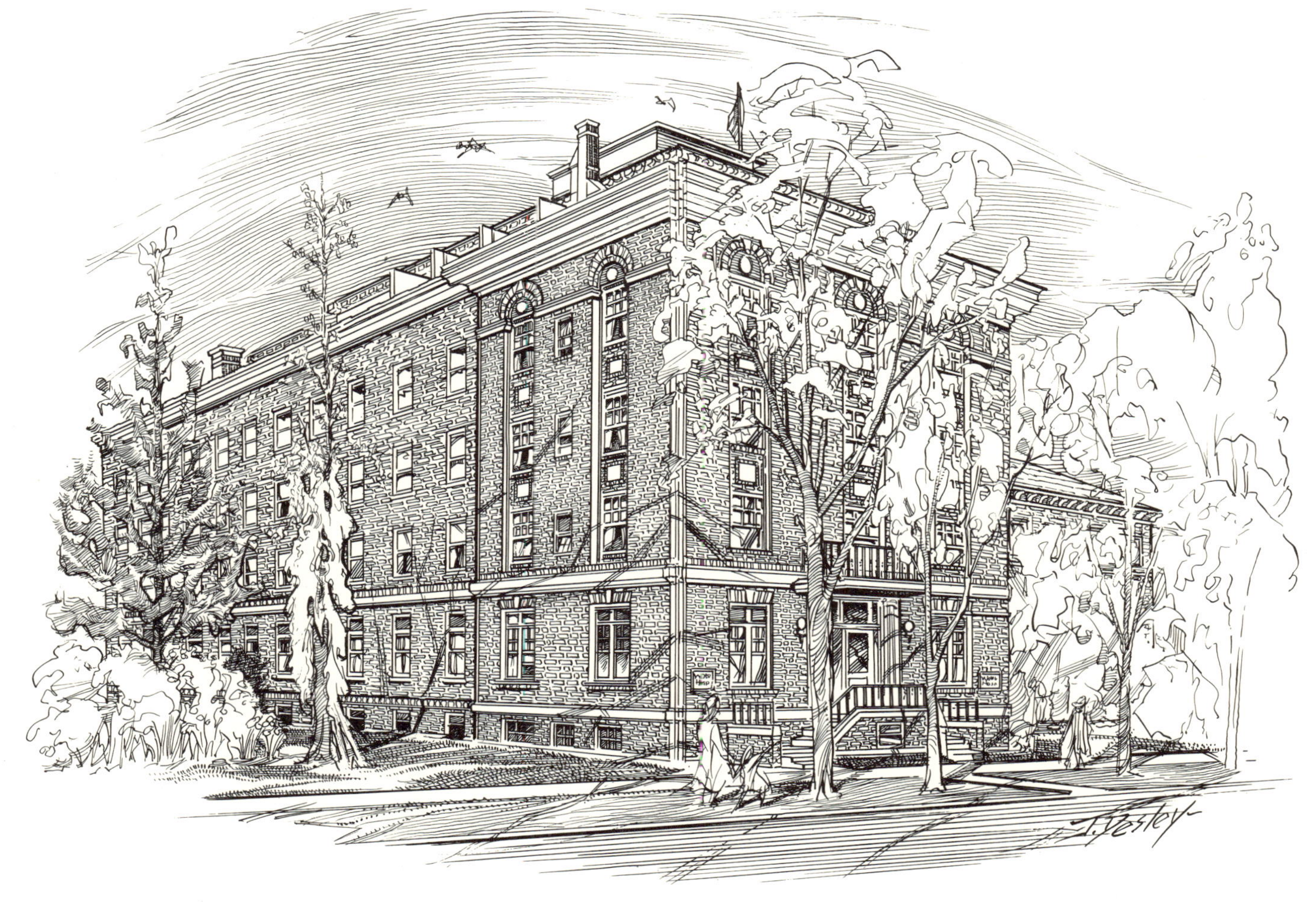

T. Pesley

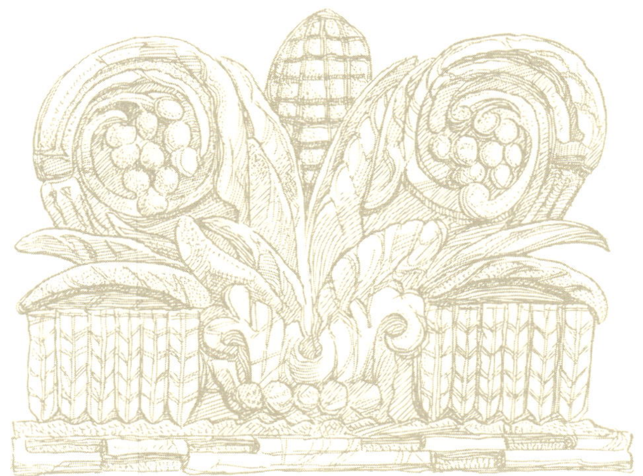

School of Physical Therapy

(Plate 29)

Initially the education annex of First Baptist Church, this unprepossessing structure, in 1970, became the home of the Mayo Clinic School of Physical Therapy. The school opened in 1938 under the direction of Dr. Frank H. Krusen, a physical medicine pioneer at Mayo. Today, the school offers a 26-month program leading to a master's degree in physical therapy through the Mayo School of Health-Related Sciences. The Baldwin Building for Community Medicine now occupies this site.

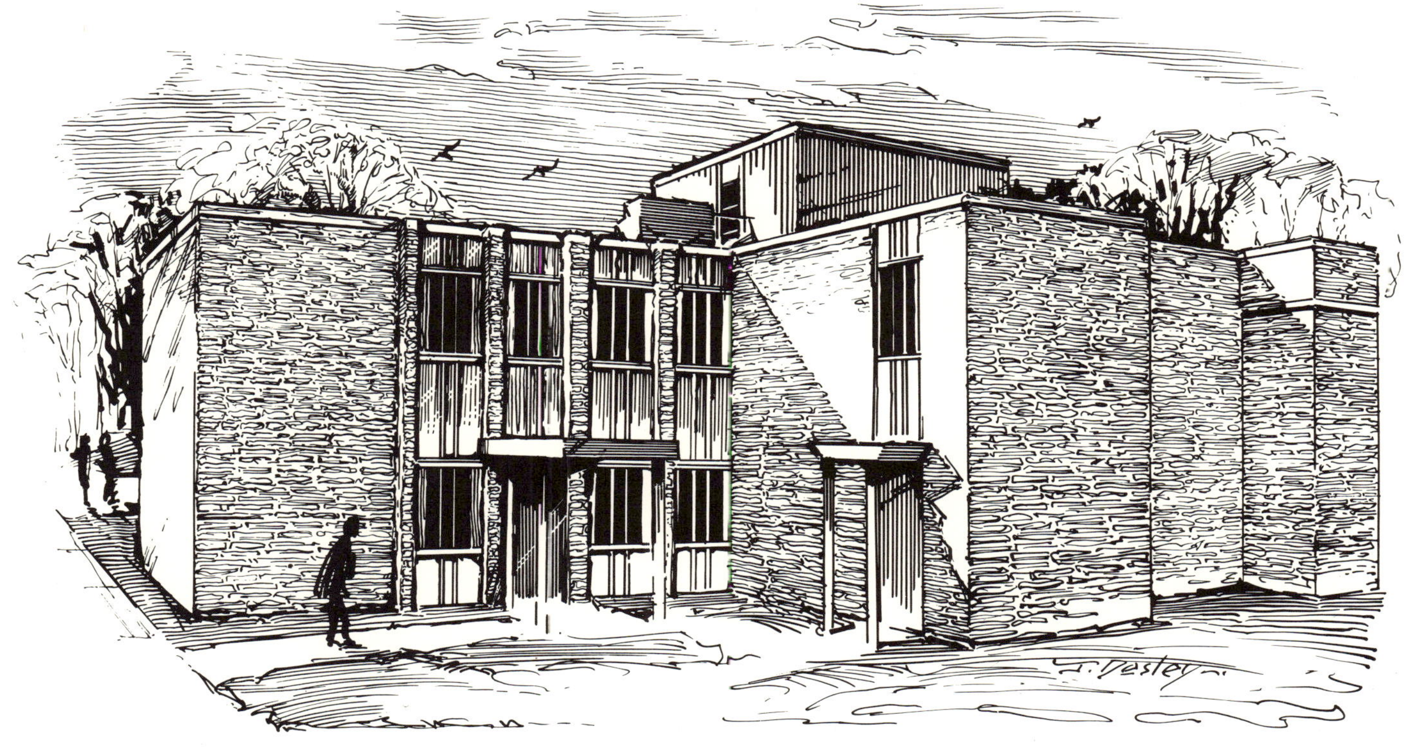

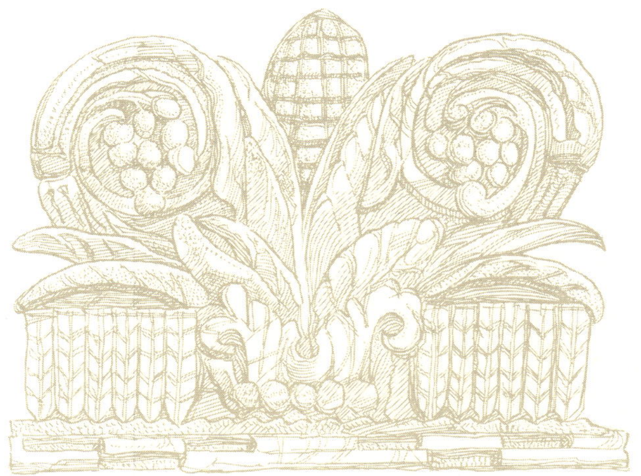

Wilson Club

(Plate 30)

The Wilson Club was a one-time hotel purchased by Mayo around 1933 for use as a housing and recreational facility for resident physicians. Rooms were available for residents, and a dining room served breakfast and lunch. A library, game rooms, a photographic darkroom, and lounge areas also were available. In 1934, the Association of Fellows named it after Dr. Louis B. Wilson, first director of the Mayo Graduate School of Medicine. The Hilton Building now occupies this site.

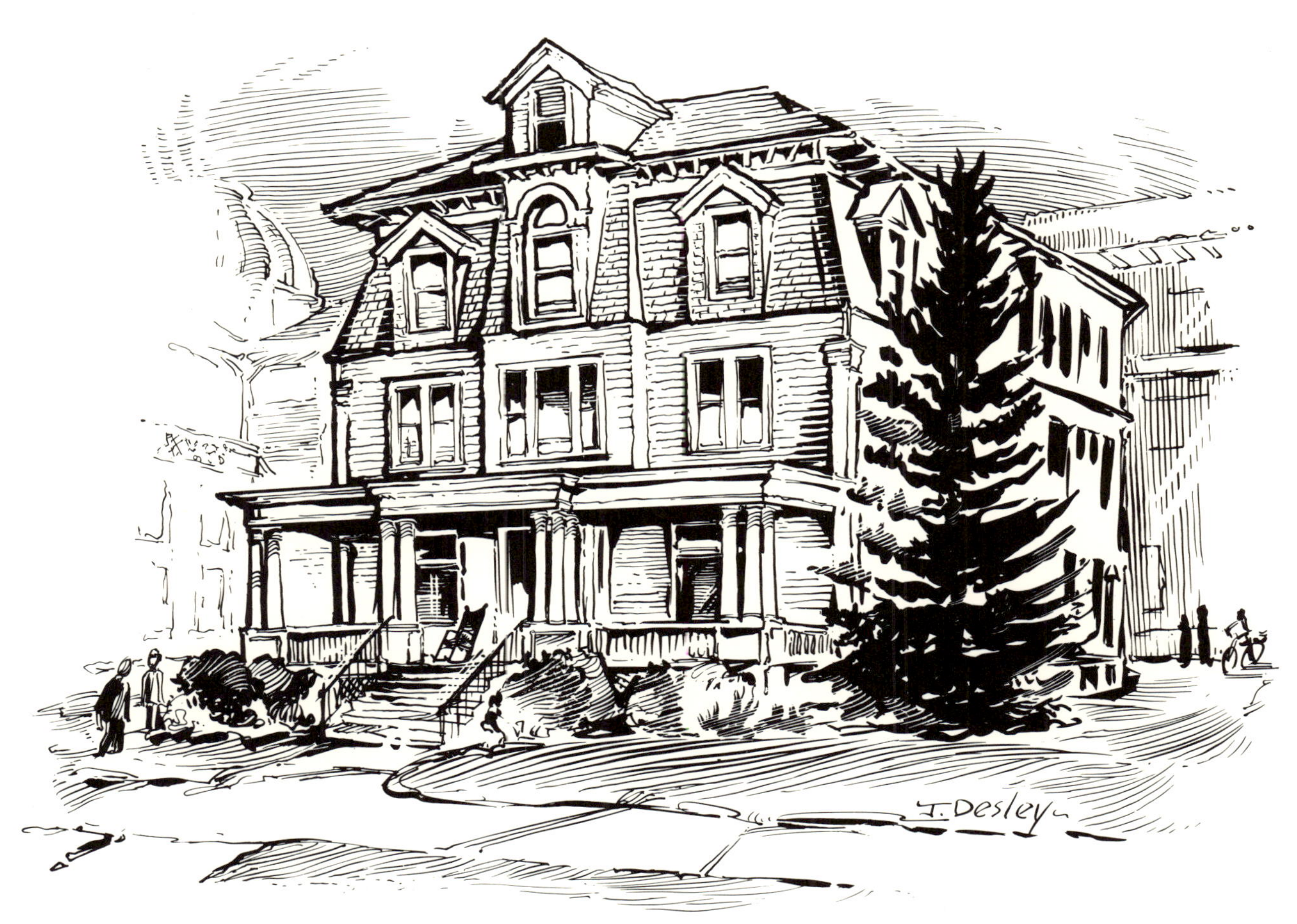
I. Desley

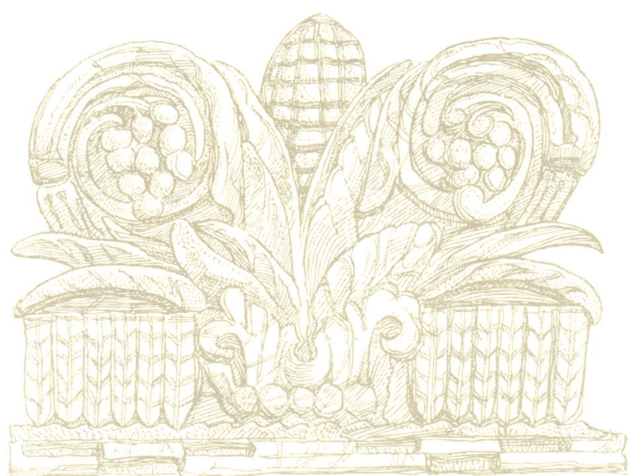

Congregational Church

(Plate 31)

Built in 1916, this Congregational Church was a familiar site to Clinic visitors and residents of Rochester for more than 50 years. The church and the Wilson Club (see page 63) were once situated across the street south of the Mayo Clinic building, on land on which the Hilton Building now stands. The structure was acquired by Mayo Foundation and used by the Physical Therapy Department in the middle and late 1960s until it was razed in 1970.

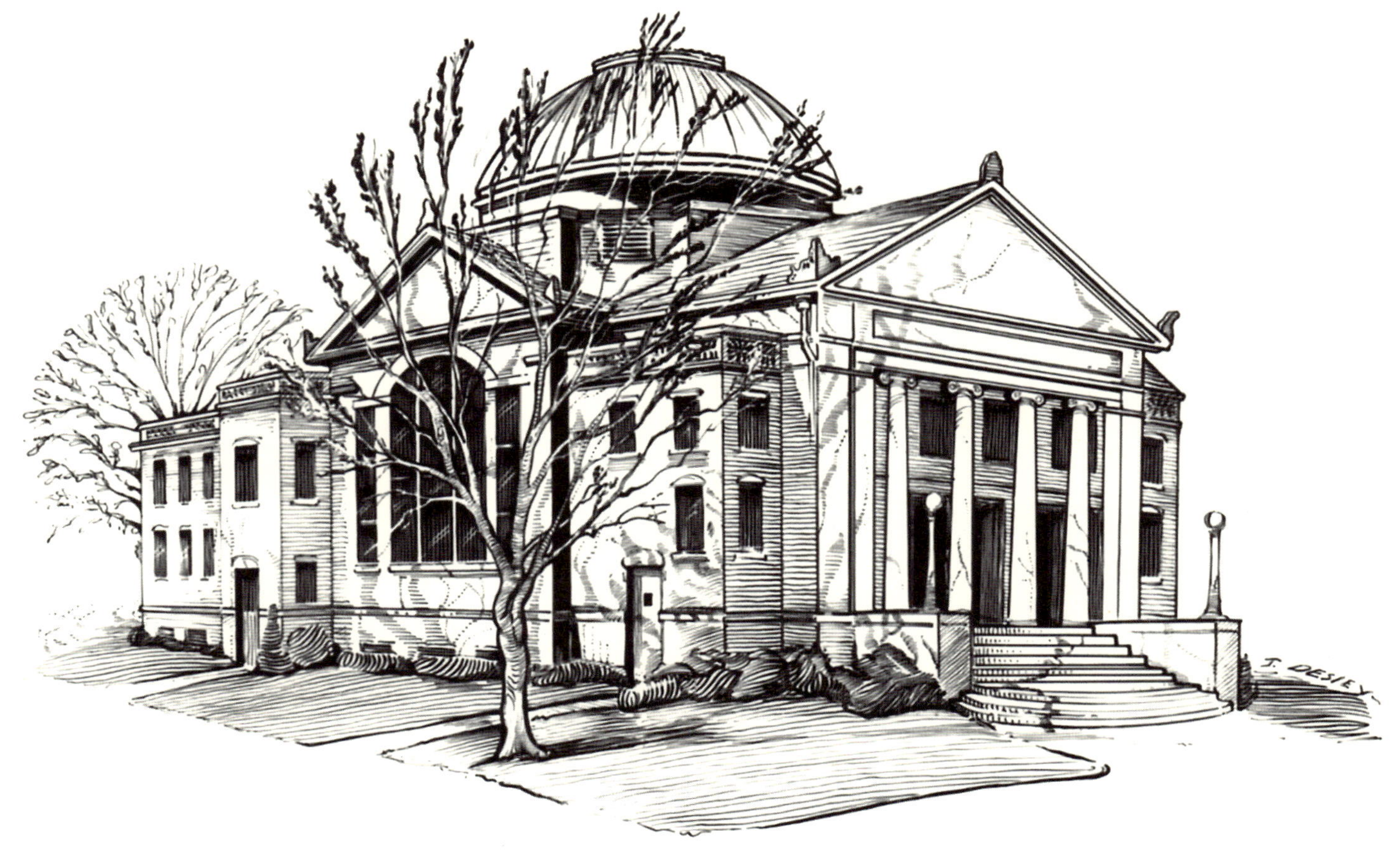

(Plate 31)

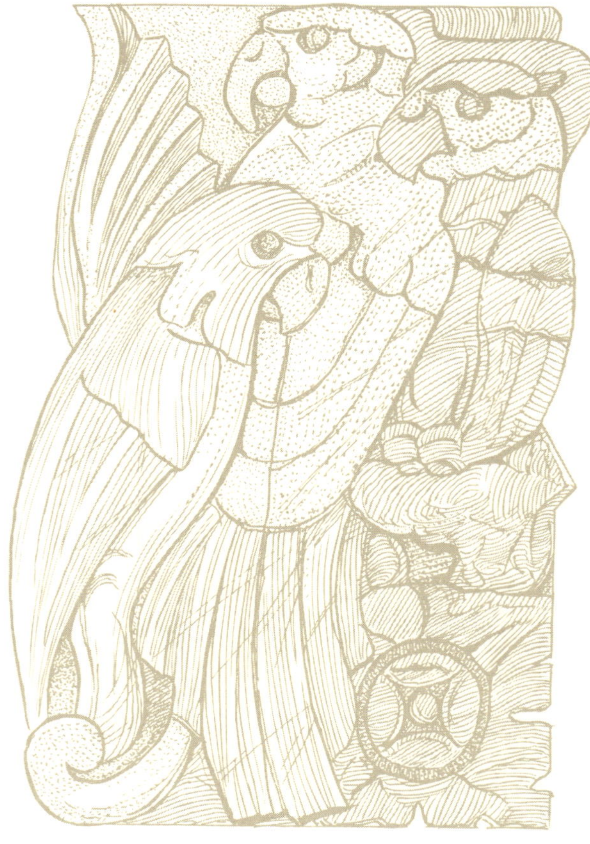

Charter House

(Plate 32)

Charter House is a full-service, continuing-care, 264-unit retirement community. Originally built by Rochester Methodist Hospital, it became part of Mayo Health System when the hospital merged with Mayo Foundation in 1986. It includes accommodations for independent and assisted living and a skilled-nursing facility. Charter House is situated at the north end of the Mayo Clinic Rochester downtown complex and is connected to Mayo by means of a carpeted, pedestrian walkway.

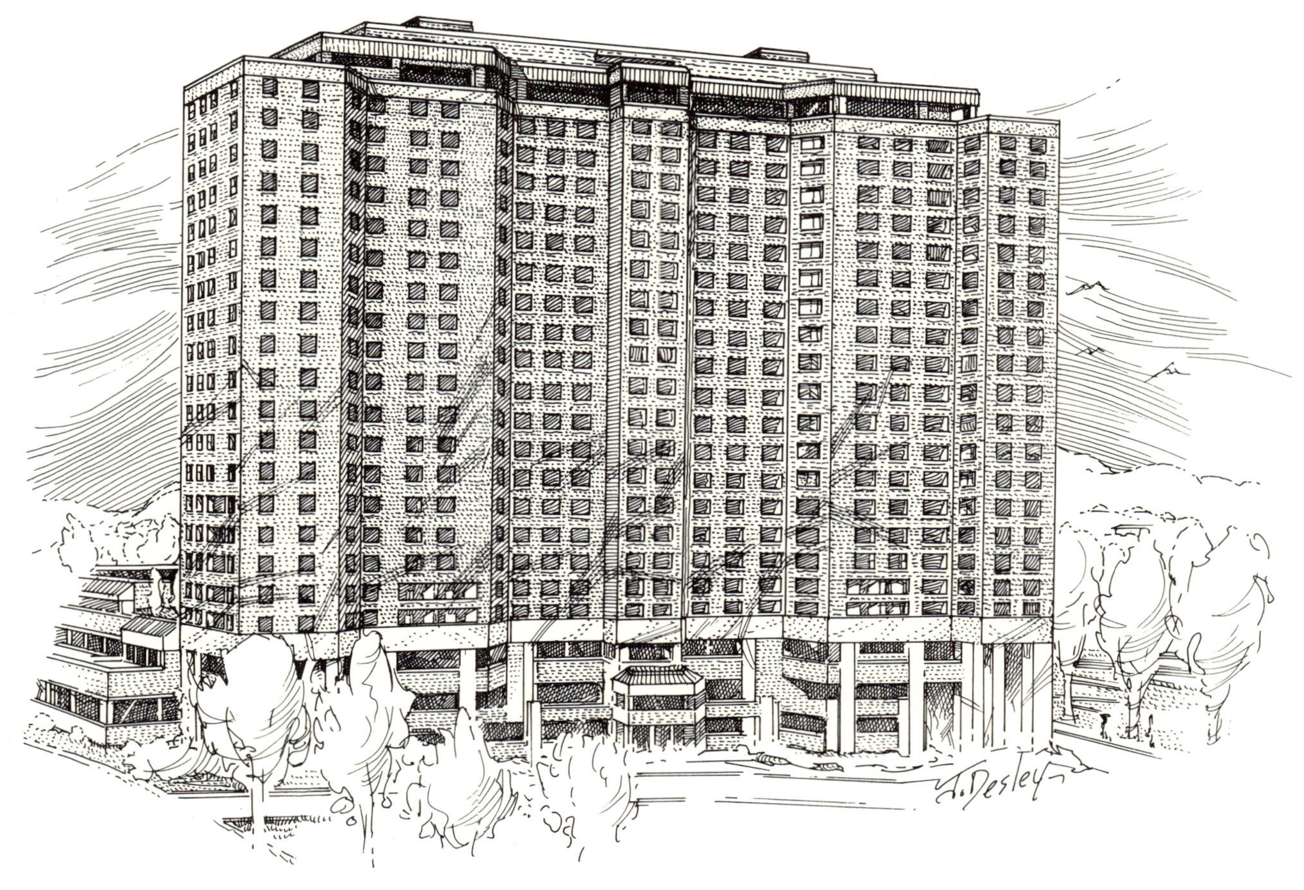

(Plate 32)

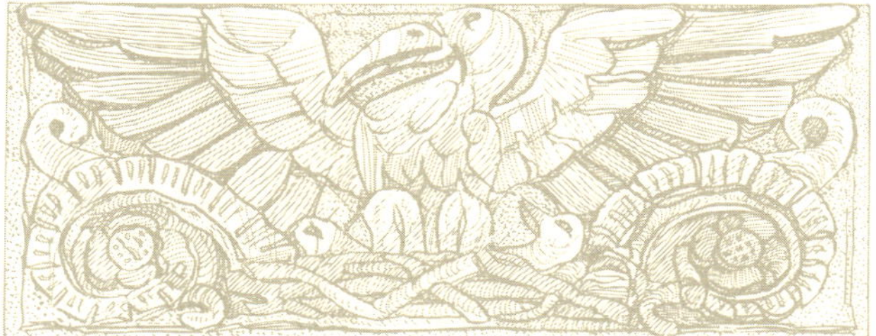

Baldwin Building

(Plate 33)

The Baldwin Building for Community Medicine was named for Mayo benefactors Jesse and Fern Baldwin, of Kearney, Nebraska. The angular structure, which was dedicated in 1987, serves as a convenient primary health care facility for Rochester area residents. It includes an urgent care center, pharmacy, and attached parking ramps for patients and staff.

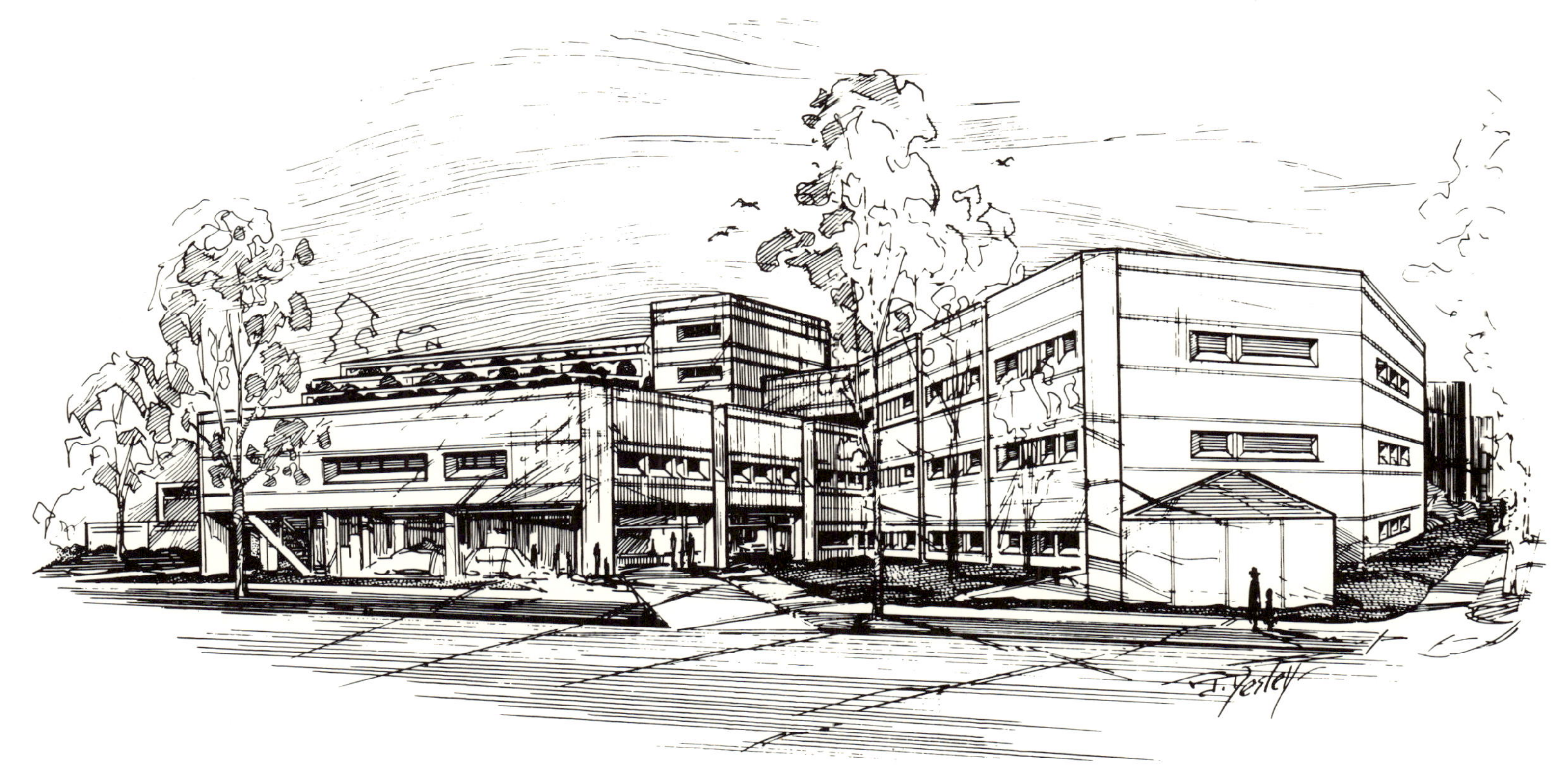

(Plate 33)

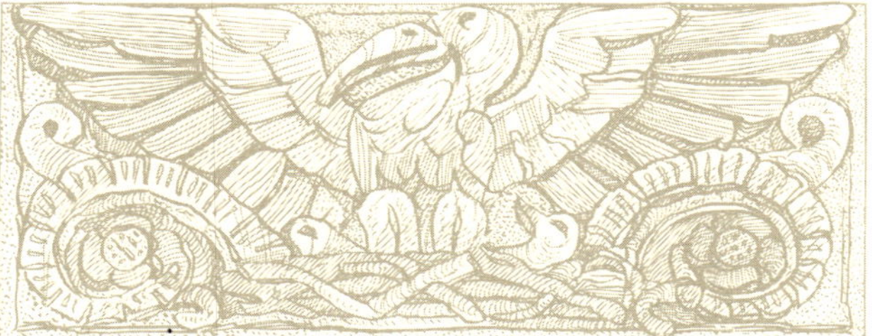

Kasson Health Facility

(Plate 34)

This 1978 drawing depicts the Kasson Health Facility in Kasson, Minnesota, then a pleasant, growing farm town of 2,000 people 15 miles west of Rochester. The building originally was owned by the city and leased to Mayo Clinic for a primary care practice in Dodge County. Over the years the town doubled in size. The facility has grown physically and in scope of medical practice. Today it is owned by Mayo Foundation. As part of the Mayo Department of Family Medicine, the Kasson Mayo Family Practice Clinic offers primary health care, easy access to specialized care at Mayo Clinic Rochester, and opportunities for residency training in family medicine.

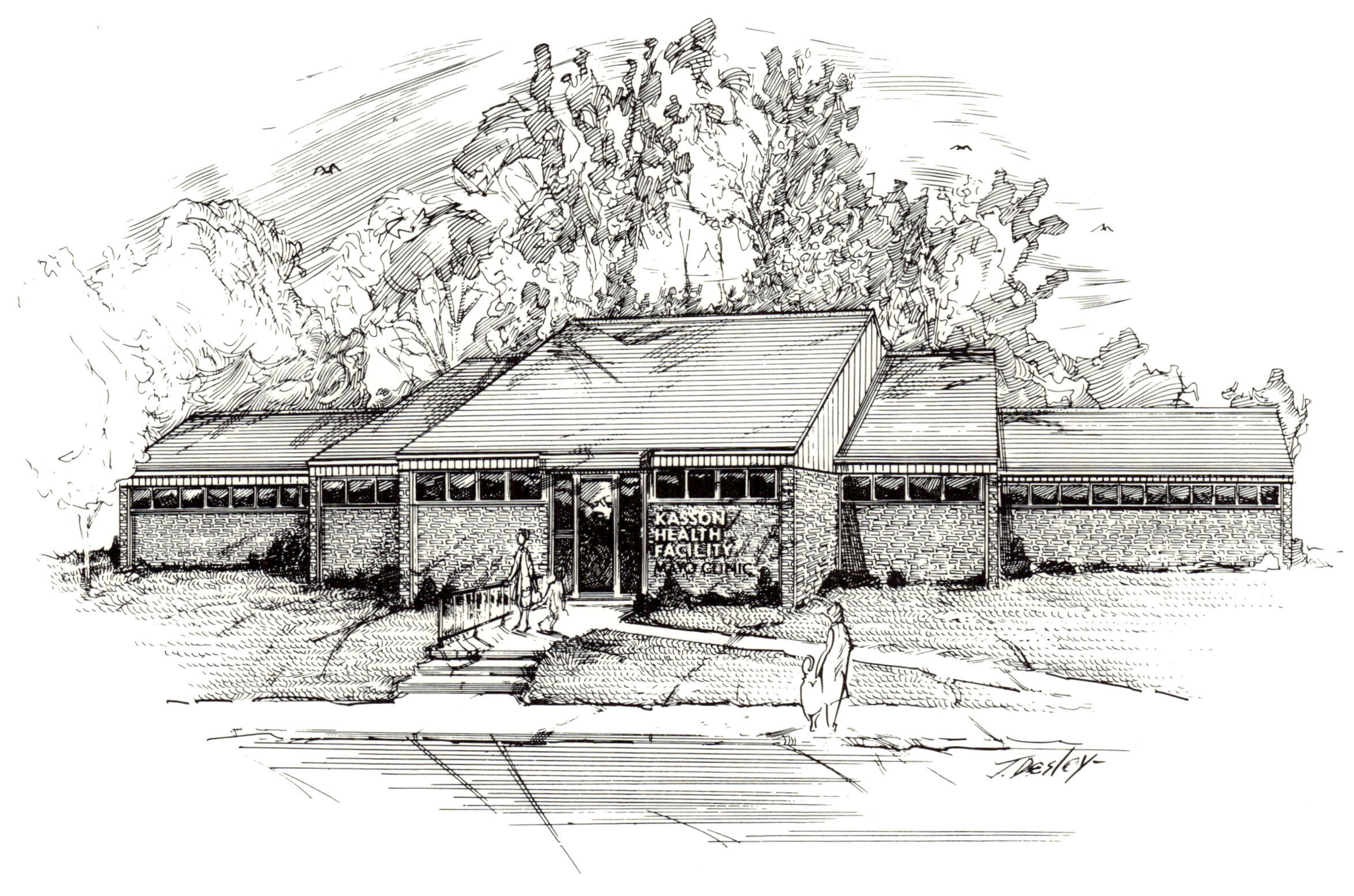
KASSON
HEALTH
FACILITY
MAYO CLINIC
T. Besley

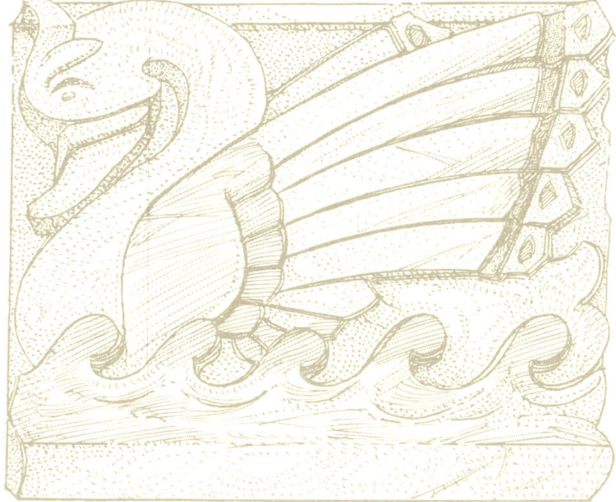

Harwick Building

(Plate 35)

The Harwick Building was named in honor of longtime Mayo administrator Harry J. Harwick. The original structure opened in 1961. In subsequent years several additions expanded the facility, including the one featured in this drawing, illustrating the design of Harry Weese Associates, of Chicago. The building includes administrative offices, employee cafeterias, and storage areas for patient medical records and X-ray films.

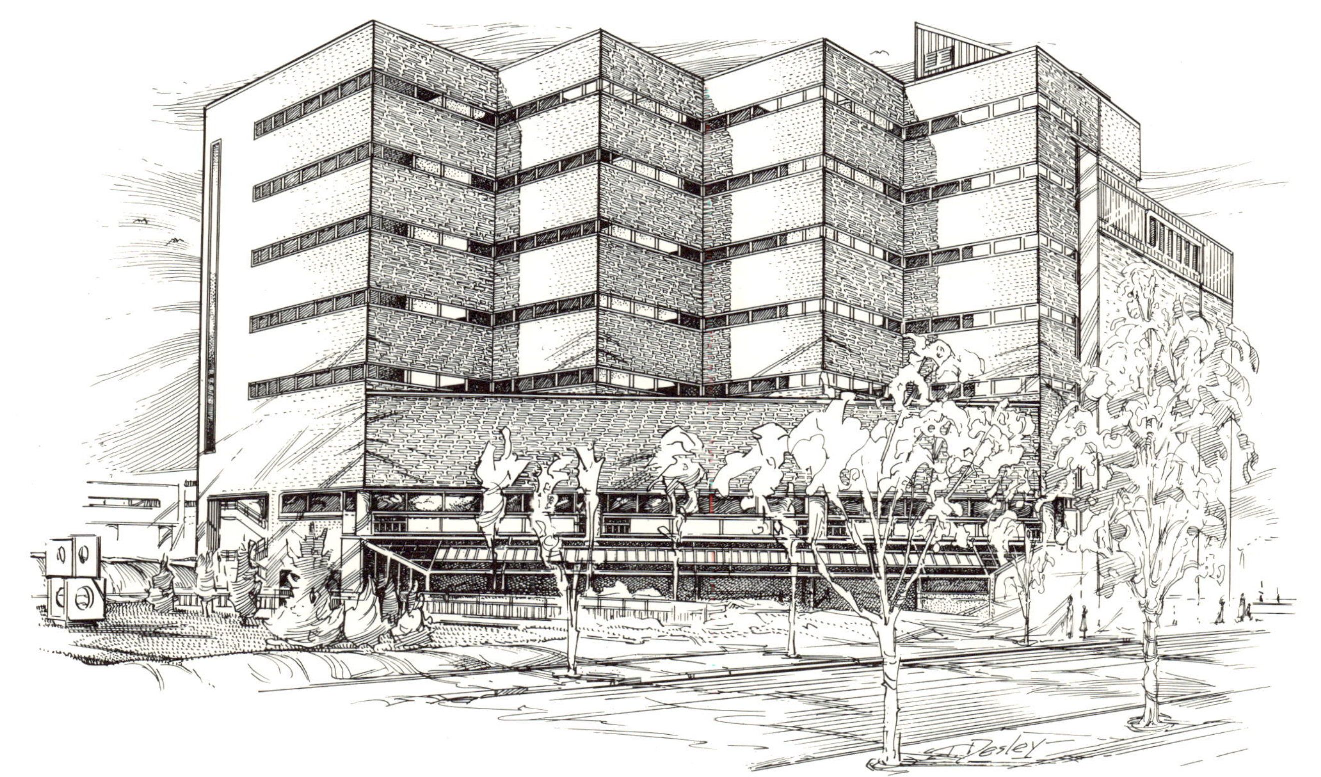

Wesley

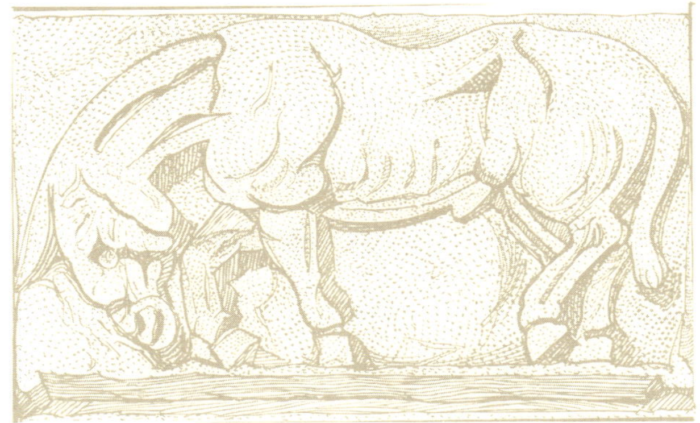

Mayo Clinic Jacksonville

(Plate 36)

Mayo Clinic Jacksonville opened in 1986 as the first major Mayo Clinic diagnostic facility outside Rochester. It is a multispecialty outpatient clinic situated in a 240-acre pine forest on the city's southeast edge. Although the focus is on specialty care, primary care programs have been added in recent years. The clinic serves a broad range of patients in Florida's "First Coast" region and beyond. The Davis Building, shown here, is named in honor of the Davis family of Jacksonville, Florida, whose pioneering philanthropy enabled Mayo to expand beyond Minnesota. The family donated the land for the clinic and spearheaded community support for Mayo in the area.

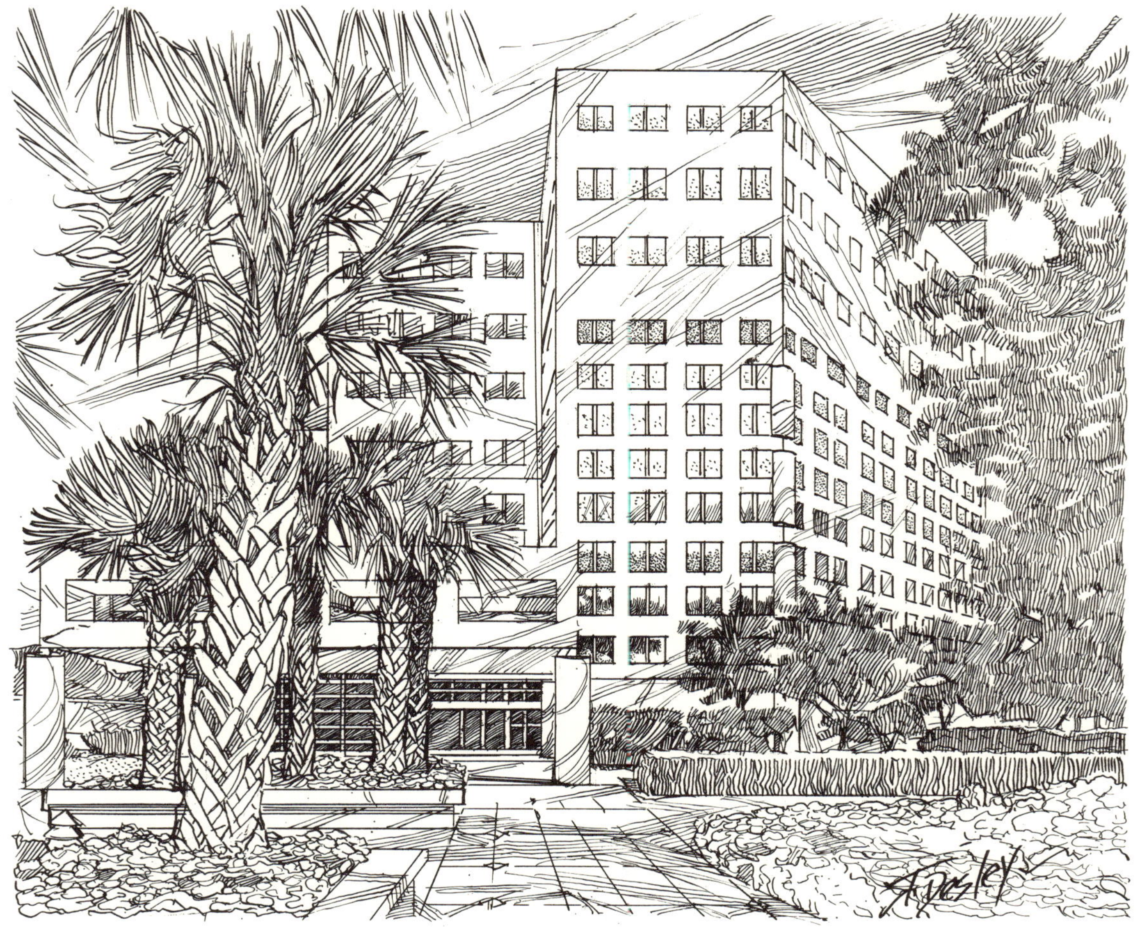

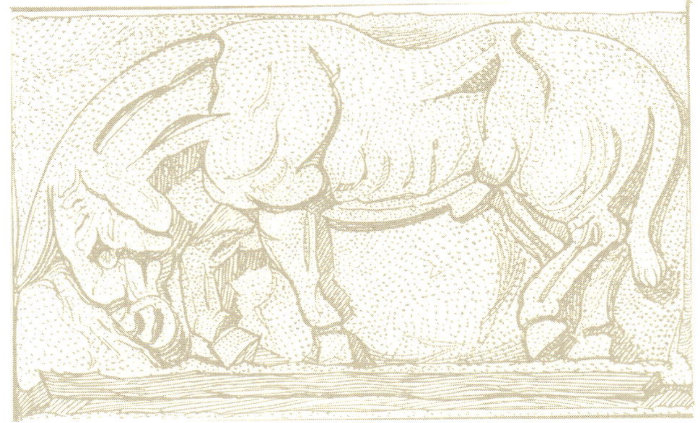

Birdsall Medical Research Building

(Plate 37)

The John H. and Jennie D. Birdsall Medical Research Building at Mayo Jacksonville houses growing programs of medical research, with special emphasis on Alzheimer's disease and other dementias. It is named in honor of Mr. and Mrs. Birdsall, of Palm Beach, Florida, for their support and interest in the advancement of medical research. Mr. Birdsall was a pioneering executive in the construction and shipping industries. The building was dedicated in 1993.

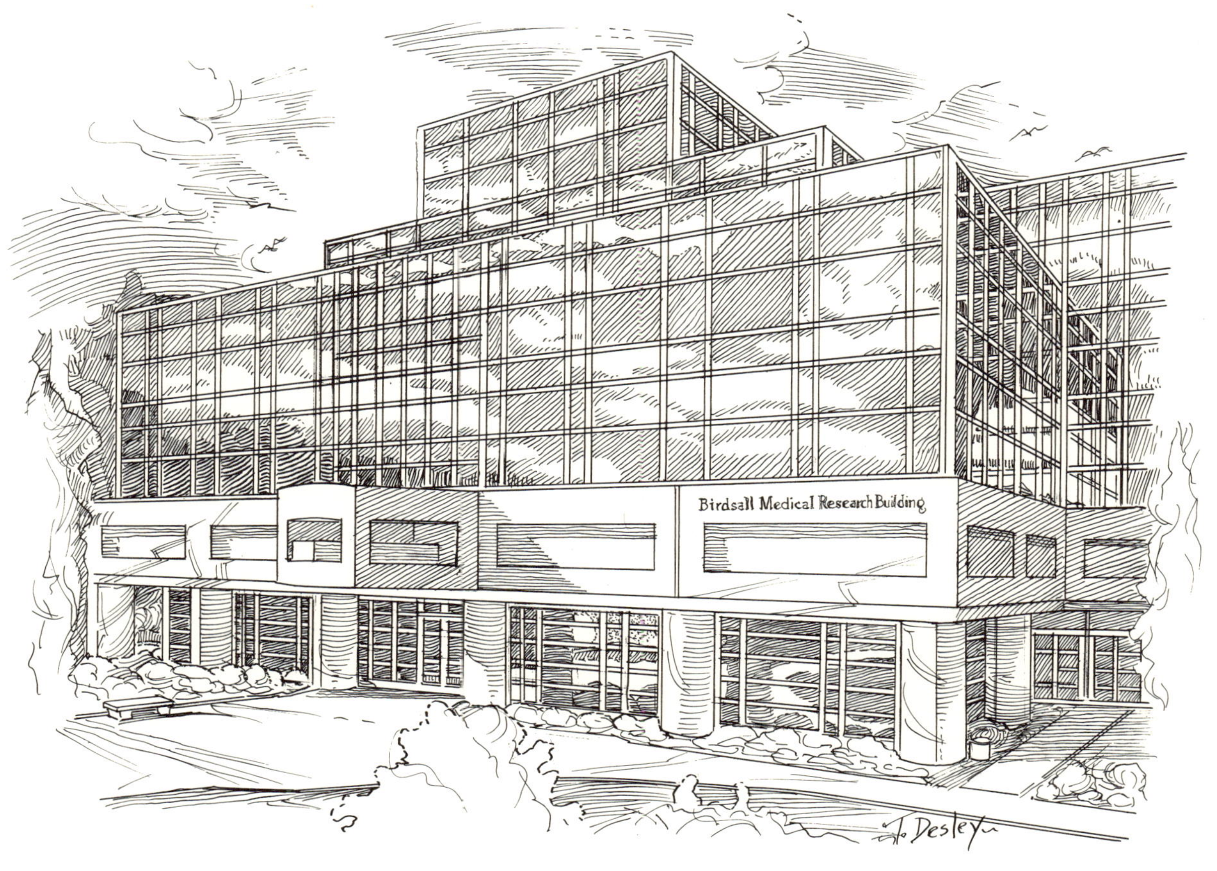
Birdsall Medical Research Building
J. Desley

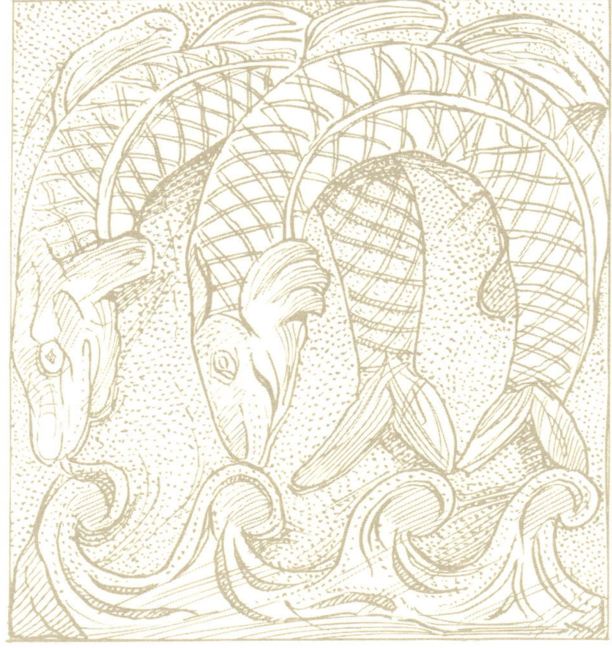

Mayo Clinic Scottsdale

(Plate 38)

Mayo Clinic Scottsdale opened in 1987. It is a multispecialty, outpatient clinic situated in the Sonoran Desert on 274 acres at the foot of the McDowell Mountains in Scottsdale. Mayo Clinic Scottsdale focuses on specialty care but also offers primary health care on site and in several offsite facilities in the surrounding area. It represents Mayo's expansion to Arizona's "Valley of the Sun."

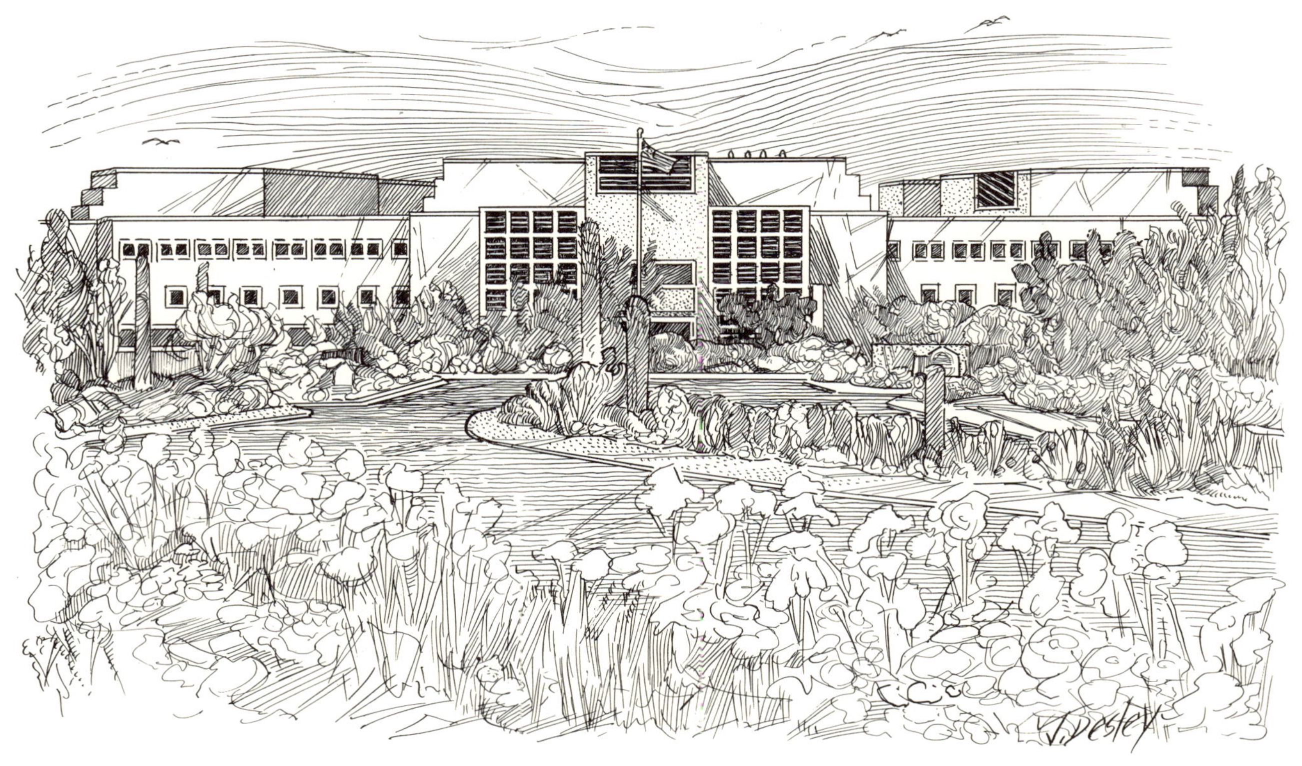

(Plate 38)

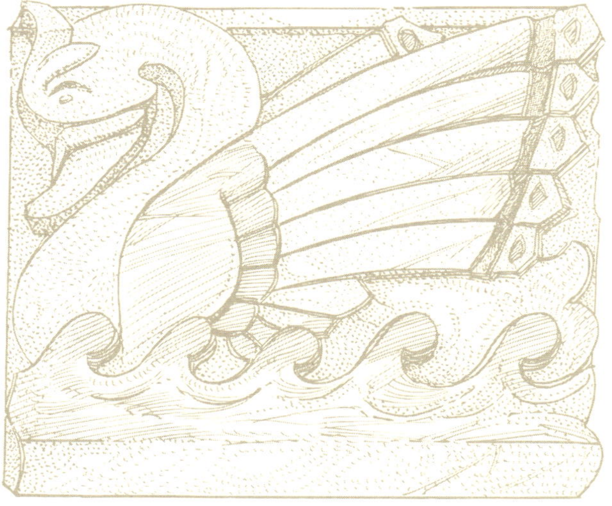

Johnson Medical Research Building

(Plate 39)

The Samuel C. Johnson Medical Research Building at Mayo Scottsdale provides quality facilities for research and honors the friendship and generosity of Samuel Johnson of Racine, Wisconsin, former chair and longest-serving public member of the Mayo Foundation Board of Trustees. The structure houses research in molecular genetics and cell and molecular biology. It opened in 1993.

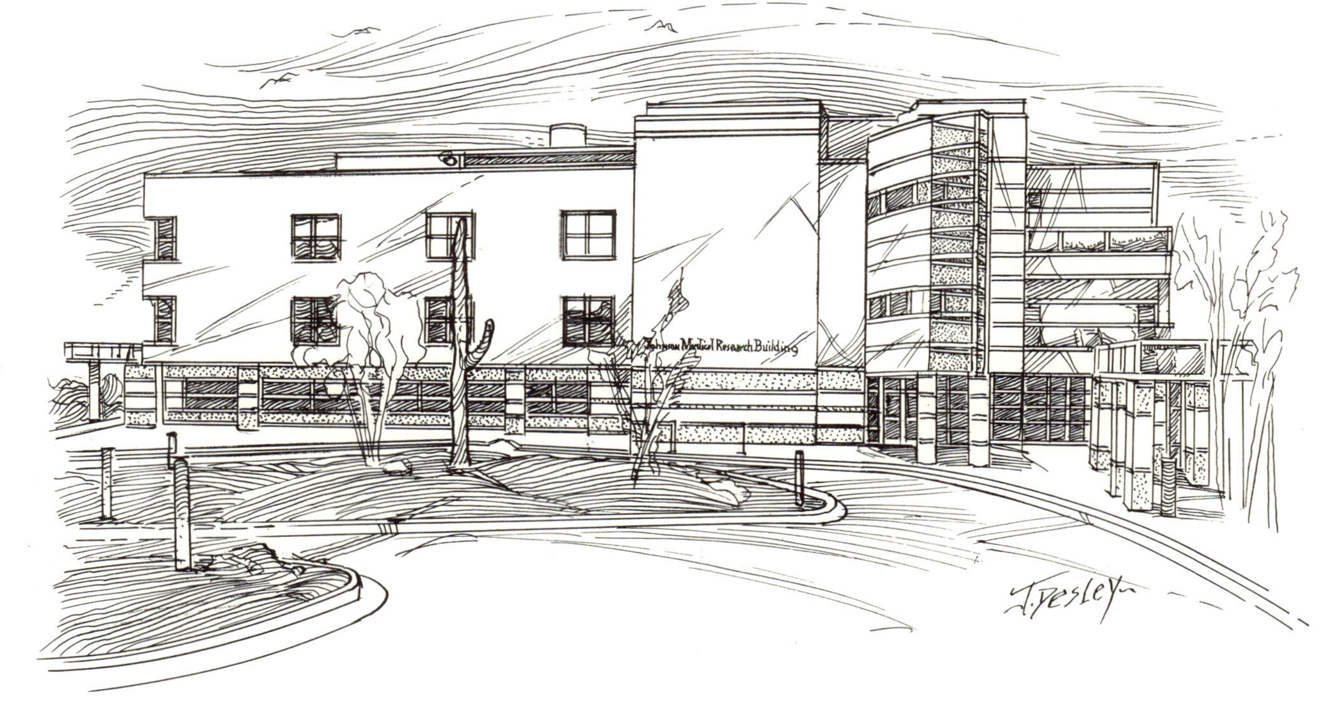
Medical Research Building